The 5 Stages of Alzheimer's

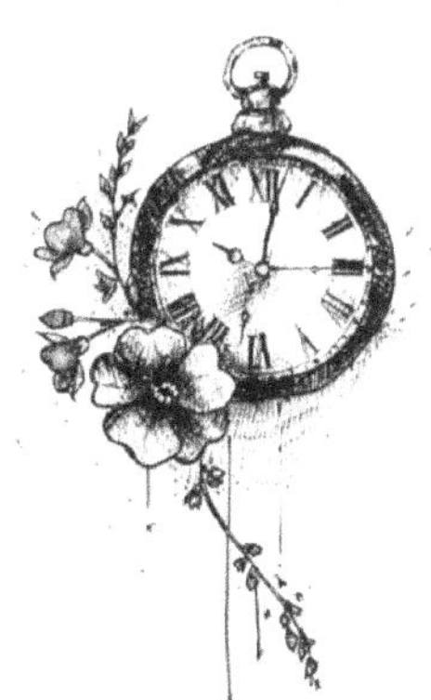

Navigate the Complexities of Caregiving,

Foster Genuine Connections with

Physical and Emotional Support

Amidst Memory and Behavioral Challenges

By G.M. Grace

Table of Contents

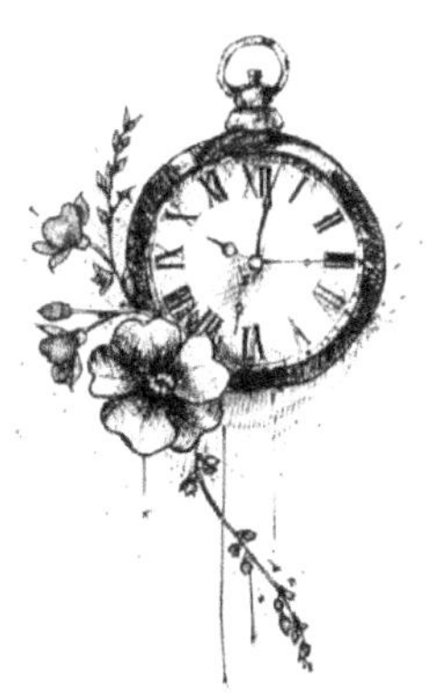

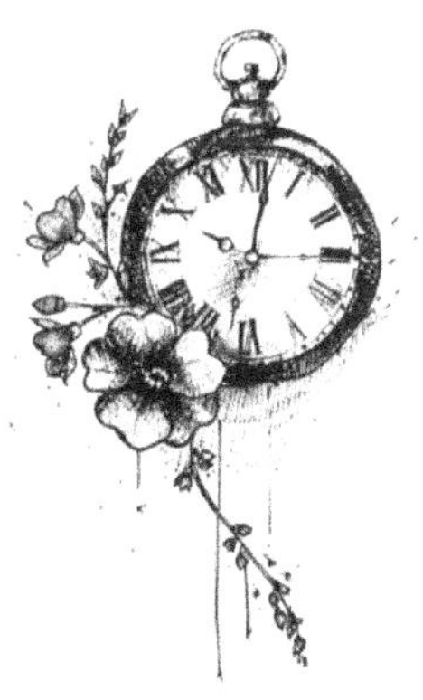

Dedication

This book is lovingly dedicated to the countless caregivers who give unselfishly of themselves daily to provide comfort, support and love to those navigating the challenging journey of Alzheimer's disease. Your dedication, strength, and compassion do not go unnoticed and are the backbone of hope and care for so many.

To my dear mother and father, who not only trained me to be their caregiver but also instilled in me the values of patience, empathy, and resilience. Your lessons have shaped my journey in ways words can hardly express, guiding me through each step with grace and wisdom.

I extend my heartfelt gratitude to my friends and family, whose unwavering support has been my anchor in stormy seas. A special thanks to Shelly, Tanya, Teresa, Gwen, and Cheri, whose kindness, understanding, and encouragement have been a source of strength and comfort. Your presence has made all the difference in both my life and the lives of those I care for.

And to my grandson, Alex, who showed me the profound impact of unconditional love through his interactions with my father. Alex, you have taught me that even amid Alzheimer's advancing stages, the simplest gestures of affection can reach through the fog, touching the heart in ways that words cannot. Your innocence and love brought my father moments of pure joy and clarity, reminding us of the powerful connection that love fosters beyond the confines of memory and cognition.

This dedication is a tribute to all of you who have been part of this journey. You have offered light in the darkest times and shown that the heart remembers what the mind may forget. Thank you for being a testament to the enduring strength of the human spirit.

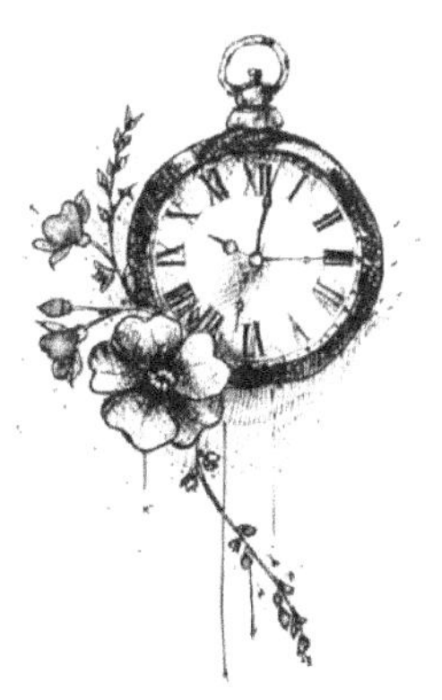

Introduction

Understanding and compassion become our most powerful tools in the face of Alzheimer's disease, a condition that weaves a complex tapestry of memory loss, cognitive decline, and emotional upheaval. This book is born out of a profound desire to offer a beacon of hope and guidance to those navigating the challenging journey of caring for a loved one with Alzheimer's. It aims to serve as a comprehensive guide, shedding light on the nuances of the disease and, more importantly, how we can care with empathy and understanding.

At the heart of this guide lies the theme of compassion and empathy. Alzheimer's disease not only affects those diagnosed with it but also has a profound impact on family members and caregivers. Through this book, we delve deeply into the importance of nurturing these qualities, recognizing them not just as moral virtues but as essential components in caring for someone with Alzheimer's. The journey through Alzheimer's is as much an emotional one as it is physical and medical, and we hope that by fostering empathy and compassion, caregivers can forge a deeper connection and understanding with their loved ones.

Crafted specifically for family members and caregivers on the front lines of this challenging battle, this book offers insights and strategies designed to equip them with the knowledge and understanding necessary to provide the best care possible. Whether you are a spouse, adult child, relative, or friend, the guidance shared within these pages is tailored to support you through the highs and lows of caregiving.

On a personal note, my desired outcome is twofold: First, to demystify Alzheimer's disease, providing readers with a clear understanding of its progression, its challenges, and the current state of research and treatment options. Second, perhaps more importantly, it is important to guide caregivers in approaching care empathetically, ensuring that their loved ones with Alzheimer's feel supported, understood, and valued at every stage of their journey.

As we embark on this exploration together, it's important to remember that you are not alone. This book is a companion for those difficult days and a reminder of the strength and love that lie at the core of caregiving. Together, we can navigate the path of Alzheimer's with grace and compassion, making each day count in the lives of those we care for and love dearly.

In addition to being a hospice volunteer and a holistic health practitioner, I bring a deeply personal perspective to this book as a caregiver who has walked the challenging path of caring for family members with both Alzheimer's and other dementias. Through firsthand experience, I have witnessed the complexities and nuances of Alzheimer's disease and caregiving, gaining valuable insights into the emotional, physical, and spiritual dimensions of this journey. This unique blend of professional expertise and personal empathy informs the compassionate approach taken in this book. My dedication to providing holistic care rooted in empathy, understanding, and dignity will shine through on every page, offering readers comfort, guidance, and inspiration as they navigate the complexities of caring for their loved ones.

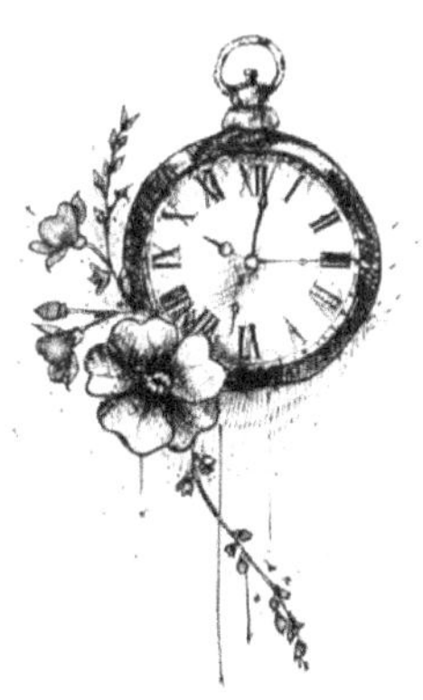

Chapter 1: Understanding Alzheimer's Disease

What is Alzheimer's Disease?

Alzheimer's disease is a progressive neurological disorder that causes the brain to shrink (atrophy) and brain cells to die. It is the most common cause of dementia, a general term for a decline in mental ability severe enough to interfere with daily life. Alzheimer's disease accounts for an estimated 60 to 80 percent of dementia cases.

The hallmark feature of Alzheimer's is the accumulation of amyloid plaques and tau tangles in the brain. This leads to disruption of communication between neurons, ultimately resulting in their death. This process begins in brain regions that control memory and other cognitive functions, leading to the early symptoms of Alzheimer's, such as forgetfulness and confusion.

As Alzheimer's advances through the brain, it leads to increasingly severe symptoms, including disorientation, mood, and behavior changes; deepening confusion about events, time, and place;

unfounded suspicions about family, friends, and professional caregivers; more severe memory loss and behavior changes; and difficulty speaking, swallowing, and walking.

Understanding Alzheimer's disease involves recognizing it as a complex condition with symptoms that can vary widely from person to person. While currently there is no cure for Alzheimer's, treatments for symptoms, combined with the proper support and interventions, can improve the quality of life for those living with the disease and their caregivers.

Causes of Alzheimer's Disease

Alzheimer's disease is a multifaceted condition whose causes encompass a combination of genetic, environmental, and lifestyle factors, all of which contribute to the progressive deterioration of the brain over time. Delving deeper into these factors reveals a complex interplay of influences:

Genetic Factors

According to the National Institute on Aging, genetic factors play a significant role in an individual's risk of developing Alzheimer's disease. Research indicates that having a parent or sibling with Alzheimer's substantially increases one's risk compared to those without a familial history of the disease. This heightened risk is attributed to the inheritance of specific genetic markers, with the APOE ε4 allele being the most well-documented genetic variant associated with an increased likelihood of developing Alzheimer's.

The APOE gene comes in several forms, but the ε4 version is particularly noteworthy for its strong correlation with Alzheimer's disease risk. However, it's important to note that inheriting this gene does not guarantee the development of Alzheimer's, but it does raise the risk compared to the general population.

In addition to the APOE ε4 allele, there are rare genetic mutations that can cause familial Alzheimer's disease, a form of early-onset Alzheimer's. These mutations are found in genes such as APP, PSEN1, and PSEN2, leading to the disease in a much smaller percentage of cases. These mutations result in the disease manifesting at a much younger age, often before 65 years of age, highlighting a direct genetic influence on the development of Alzheimer's.

Overall, the interplay between genetics and family history in Alzheimer's disease underscores the importance of genetic research in understanding and potentially mitigating the risk of developing this debilitating condition.

Environmental and Lifestyle Factors:

Age: Advancing age is indeed the most significant risk factor for Alzheimer's disease, with studies showing that the risk of developing Alzheimer's doubles approximately every five years after the age of 65. This correlation highlights that while aging itself does not directly cause Alzheimer's, the process of aging increases the vulnerability to the disease. The mechanisms behind this increased risk are complex and multifaceted, involving changes in brain structure and function alongside a decline in the brain's ability to repair itself. This susceptibility is further compounded by the presence of other risk factors that often accompany aging, such as cardiovascular disease, diabetes, and hypertension, which can exacerbate the risk of developing Alzheimer's. Moreover, lifestyle factors, including physical inactivity, obesity, and smoking, which are more prevalent or consequential in later life, also contribute significantly to the risk profile for Alzheimer's disease. Thus, aging acts as a backdrop against which these other risk factors may either emerge or worsen, cumulatively increasing the likelihood of Alzheimer's disease as individuals grow old.

Heart-Health Risk Factors: Several risk factors associated with cardiovascular health, including hypertension, high cholesterol, diabetes, and obesity, are also implicated in the development of Alzheimer's disease and vascular dementia. These conditions contribute to vascular changes and disruptions in blood flow to the brain, exacerbating cognitive decline.

Head Trauma: Severe head injuries, including traumatic brain injuries (TBI) from accidents or sports-related concussions, have been identified as significant risk factors for the development of Alzheimer's disease in later life. Studies suggest that moderate to severe TBI is associated with an increased risk of Alzheimer's, mainly when the injury involves loss of consciousness (LOC). Research indicates that not all cases of TBI lead to Alzheimer's, but the risk is notably higher in moderate and severe cases of head injury.

The connection between head trauma and Alzheimer's disease is believed to be biologically plausible, as head injuries can lead to the over-expression of beta-amyloid precursor proteins, which are key components in the pathogenesis of Alzheimer's disease. This over-expression can result in the accumulation of abnormal protein aggregates, known as amyloid plaques, characteristic of Alzheimer's. Additionally, direct damage to the brain tissue during the injury and subsequent neuroinflammatory responses may further contribute to the development of Alzheimer's disease. The exact mechanisms linking TBI to Alzheimer's are still a subject of ongoing research, with proposed theories including the disruption of neural pathways and enhanced vulnerability to neurodegeneration.

Brain Changes

Plaques and Tangles: In Alzheimer's disease, two primary pathological hallmarks are observed in the brain: the accumulation of beta-amyloid plaques and tau protein tangles. Beta-amyloid plaques form when protein pieces called beta-amyloid, which come from a more significant protein found in the fatty membrane surrounding nerve cells, clump together. These plaques accumulate outside neurons and disrupt cell function by interfering with neuronal communication.

Tau protein tangles, on the other hand, occur inside neurons. Tau proteins play a crucial role in maintaining the structure of neurons. However, in Alzheimer's disease, these proteins become abnormally phosphorylated and form tangles, which lead to the collapse of the neuron's transport system. This disruption results in the malfunction and death of nerve cells, contributing significantly to the cognitive decline seen in Alzheimer's patients.

These changes—beta-amyloid plaques and tau tangles—hinder neuronal communication and trigger a cascade of neurodegenerative processes, including inflammation and further cellular damage, leading to the progressive symptoms of Alzheimer's disease.

This damage progresses over time, leading to widespread neuronal dysfunction and death. Consequently, the loss of neurons in key brain regions responsible for memory, cognition, and other functions results in the progressive symptoms of Alzheimer's disease, including memory loss, confusion, and eventual loss of bodily functions. Understanding these mechanisms is crucial for developing therapeutic strategies aimed at mitigating the progression of Alzheimer's disease.

Other Possible Factors

Education, Social Engagement, and Brain-Active Activities: Education, social engagement, and brain-active activities are potential protective factors against Alzheimer's disease. Research indicates that participating in intellectually stimulating tasks, maintaining an active social life, and pursuing higher levels of education may help build cognitive reserve. Cognitive reserve refers to the brain's ability to withstand damage and function typically despite pathology. Individuals may develop more robust neural networks by engaging in these activities, which can offset the impact of Alzheimer 's-related changes and delay symptom onset. While these factors do not guarantee immunity from the disease, they are associated with a reduced risk and may contribute to overall brain health.

Diet and Exercise: While ongoing research explores the impact of diet and exercise on Alzheimer's risk, evidence suggests that adopting a healthy lifestyle, including a balanced diet and regular physical activity, may help reduce susceptibility to the disease. These lifestyle factors promote cardiovascular health, reduce inflammation, and support brain function.

Sleep Patterns: UC Berkeley research has shown a compelling association between disrupted sleep patterns and a heightened risk of developing Alzheimer's disease. Specifically, individuals experiencing difficulties falling asleep and maintaining sleep continuity are more vulnerable. Studies indicate that disturbances in sleep-wake cycles, characterized by fragmented sleep or insomnia symptoms, may contribute to the onset or progression of Alzheimer's. These sleep disruptions potentially disrupt the brain's ability to clear harmful proteins, such as beta-amyloid and tau, which are hallmark features of Alzheimer's pathology. Additionally, inadequate sleep may impair cognitive function and exacerbate neuroinflammation, both of which are implicated in the development of Alzheimer's disease. Therefore, optimizing sleep quality and addressing sleep-related issues may represent a valuable strategy for mitigating the risk or delaying the progression of Alzheimer's disease.

Other Factors

Sex: Research indicates that women have a higher likelihood of developing Alzheimer's disease compared to men, potentially attributed to their longer life expectancies.

Depression: Additionally, individuals with a history of depression may face an increased risk of Alzheimer's disease, though further studies are needed to understand this association fully.

It's important to note that having one or even multiple risk factors does not guarantee that a person will develop Alzheimer's disease. Conversely, the absence of risk factors does not ensure that a person will be free from the disease. However, understanding these factors can guide lifestyle choices and healthcare strategies to potentially lower the risk or delay the onset of Alzheimer's. Understanding the complex interplay of genetic, environmental, and lifestyle factors underlying Alzheimer's disease is essential for developing effective prevention strategies and treatment options. Ongoing research efforts aim to unravel the intricacies of these causes, paving the way for more targeted interventions to combat or delay the onset of Alzheimer's disease and improve outcomes for affected individuals and their families.

Five Stages of Alzheimer's Disease

Alzheimer's disease typically progresses through five stages, each characterized by specific symptoms and changes in cognitive and functional abilities. These stages provide insights into the disease's gradual evolution and impact on individuals and their families.

Stage 1: Preclinical Alzheimer's Disease

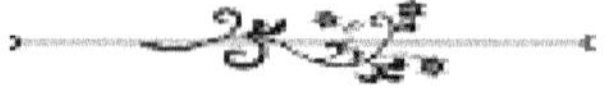

The subtle shifts began in the soft, diffused light of early autumn. My father, a man of sharp wit and boundless energy, started to misplace the familiar – keys, glasses, and even the names of old friends seemed to slip through his grasp like water. At first, these moments were like whispers in a crowded room, easy to dismiss amidst the noise of daily life. But as the leaves turned from green to gold, so too did the nature of our reality.

I remember the day it became impossible to ignore. We sat in his study, a room lined with books and memories, discussing plans for my upcoming birthday. Mid-conversation, he paused, his brow furrowed in confusion. "What were we talking about, again?" he asked, a hint of frustration in his voice. It was a small moment, but it echoed loudly in the silence that followed.

Determined to find answers, we embarked on a journey that led us to doctors' offices and specialists' rooms, each visit a step toward understanding. The diagnosis of Stage 1 Alzheimer's disease came as a whisper turned into a shout, changing the melody of our lives.

In those early days, I became a student of patience and empathy. I learned the importance of living in the moment, cherishing the clarity when it came, and offering support when it waned. We developed strategies and simple adjustments to daily life that became beacons of hope. A shared calendar for important dates, labels on cabinets, and gentle reminders of names and places became threads in the fabric of our new normal.

Despite the diagnosis, we found moments of joy and laughter. I would tell him stories from my childhood, and he would listen, his eyes lighting up with recognition and delight. Sometimes, he would share his memories, tales from his youth that seemed untouched by the fog of Alzheimer's. In these moments, I saw not just my father but the man he had always been – strong, kind, and endlessly curious.

We walked in the evenings, the setting sun casting long shadows on the path ahead. During these walks, we spoke of fears and hopes for the future. He expressed his worries about becoming a burden, about the spaces in his memory that seemed to grow wider each day. I held his hand, offering assurances not just of my love but of my unwavering support, no matter what lay ahead.

As we navigated the complexities of Stage 1 Alzheimer's, I became his anchor, just as he had been mine throughout my life. We learned to communicate in new ways, finding comfort in shared silences and understanding the space between words. Though uninvited, the disease brought a deeper connection, a reminder of the enduring strength of love and family.

The journey through Alzheimer's is one of unpredictable twists and turns, but it is also a testament to the resilience of the human spirit. My father, with his gentle courage and quiet determination, taught me that even in the face of change, there is beauty to be found in the act of caring and strength in the bonds that hold us together.

As the seasons changed, we stood together, a father and his daughter, ready to face whatever came our way with grace and love. In the whispers of change, we found not just challenge but opportunity – the chance to grow closer, understand more profoundly, and love more fully than we ever thought possible.

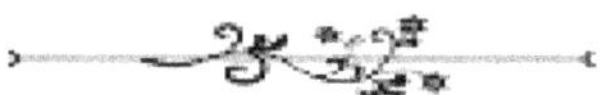

In the initial stage of Alzheimer's disease, known as preclinical Alzheimer's disease, individuals do not exhibit any noticeable symptoms, yet significant changes are occurring in their brains. Here are the key points to understand about this stage:

Characteristics

Absence of Symptoms: As already mentioned, the initial stage of Alzheimer's disease is characterized by an absence of noticeable cognitive or functional symptoms. During this period, individuals can maintain their daily routines and activities without apparent difficulty, and no significant impairments in memory, communication, or reasoning are observable to others. This stage can be particularly challenging to identify because the individual appears to function normally, and there are no outward signs indicating the onset of Alzheimer's.

Despite the lack of visible symptoms, it's crucial to understand that significant changes are already occurring within the brain. At the cellular and molecular levels, alterations are taking place that will eventually lead to the symptoms commonly associated with Alzheimer's disease. These changes involve the accumulation of amyloid-beta plaques and tau tangles, which disrupt communication between neurons and lead to cell death. This period of preclinical Alzheimer's, where changes are happening internally without affecting the individual's external behavior or capabilities, underscores the complexity of the disease and the challenge of early detection.

Recognizing this silent phase is essential for researchers and healthcare professionals as it offers a potential window for intervention before the onset of symptoms. Understanding the mechanisms and markers of this early stage is the focus of ongoing research, aiming to develop strategies for early detection, prevention, and, ultimately, treatments that could delay or halt the progression of Alzheimer's disease. Even though individuals in this stage do not exhibit symptoms, awareness of the disease's covert progression is a critical step in addressing Alzheimer's comprehensively.

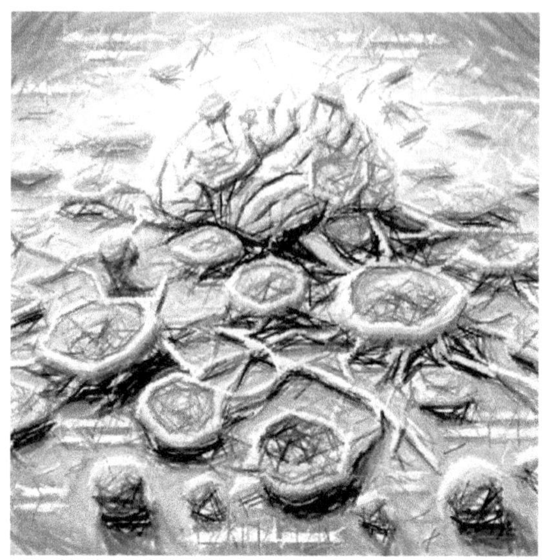

The presence of both amyloid plaques and tau tangles are key contributors to the gradual decline in cognitive function seen in Alzheimer's disease. As these abnormal proteins accumulate, they initiate a cascade of neural damage and brain atrophy, particularly affecting brain regions involved in memory, reasoning, and complex thought processes. The interplay between amyloid plaques and tau tangles is a focus of ongoing research, as understanding their precise roles and interactions could lead to the development of targeted treatments for Alzheimer's disease.

Duration: The duration of preclinical Alzheimer's disease is one of its most intriguing and challenging aspects, as this stage can persist for years or even decades before any observable symptoms emerge. This prolonged period of asymptomatic progression underscores the complexity of Alzheimer's disease and highlights the importance of early detection and intervention.

Researchers are deeply invested in studying this preclinical stage to identify early disease markers. These markers could be biochemical, genetic, or observable through advanced imaging techniques. Identifying such markers is critical for developing interventions that may delay or prevent the progression of symptomatic Alzheimer's disease. Early interventions could target the biochemical processes underlying the accumulation of amyloid plaques and tau tangles, thereby slowing down or halting the disease's progression before cognitive decline begins.

Understanding preclinical Alzheimer's disease is crucial for several reasons. Firstly, it provides a window of opportunity for early detection, essential for any potential intervention to be most effective. Secondly, by identifying individuals at this stage, researchers can explore strategies to slow down or mitigate the disease's impact on cognition and quality of life. These strategies could include lifestyle changes, pharmacological interventions, or a combination of approaches to preserve brain health and function.

Let's delve deeper into the diagnostic evaluations during the preclinical stage of Alzheimer's disease:

Diagnostic Evaluations: During this stage, individuals may undergo several assessments and screenings to detect early signs of Alzheimer's disease. These evaluations are crucial for identifying subtle changes in the brain before noticeable symptoms emerge.

Here are two key diagnostic approaches:

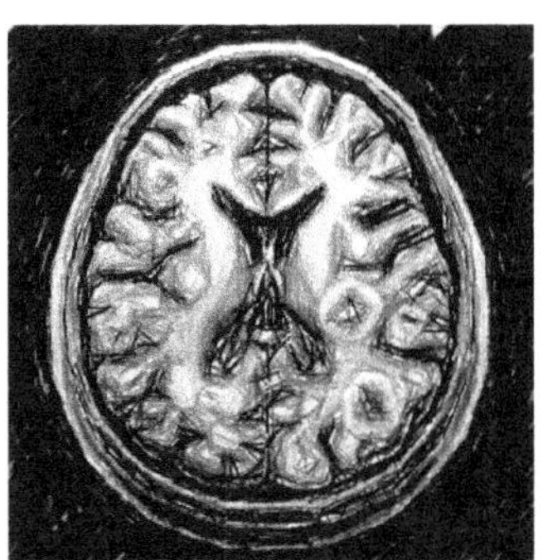

Neuroimaging Techniques

Positron Emission Tomography (PET) Scans: Neuroimaging techniques, particularly Positron Emission Tomography (PET) scans, play a pivotal role in the study and early detection of Alzheimer's disease, especially during its preclinical stages. PET scans are advanced imaging modalities that enable the visualization of specific molecular processes within the brain, offering unique insights into the onset and progression of neurological conditions like Alzheimer's.

In preclinical Alzheimer's, PET scans are primarily used to detect the presence of amyloid plaques. The technique involves injecting a radioactive tracer into the bloodstream, designed to bind specifically to amyloid proteins. As the tracer circulates through the brain, it attaches to any amyloid plaques present, making them visible on the PET scan.

The ability of PET scans to reveal the distribution and density of amyloid plaques in the brain is invaluable for early detection efforts. By identifying amyloid accumulation before the onset of clinical symptoms, PET scans help to identify individuals at risk for developing symptomatic Alzheimer's disease.

The use of PET scans in detecting amyloid plaques represents a significant advancement in Alzheimer's research, providing a powerful tool for understanding the disease's early stages. Through these imaging techniques, researchers and clinicians can gain a deeper understanding of the pathological changes occurring in the brain, opening the door to targeted interventions that could alter the course of Alzheimer's disease for those at risk.

Biomarker Analyses

Cerebrospinal Fluid (CSF) Analysis: Biomarker analyses, such as Cerebrospinal Fluid (CSF) analysis, offer another critical avenue for early detection and understanding Alzheimer's pathology. CSF surrounds the brain and spinal cord, providing essential nutrients and acting as a protective cushion. By analyzing CSF samples, researchers can detect specific biomarkers associated with Alzheimer's disease. Key biomarkers include Amyloid-beta (Aβ), where elevated levels in the CSF correlate with amyloid plaque deposition in the brain; Tau Protein, with increased levels indicating neurodegeneration and the presence of tau tangles; and Phosphorylated Tau (p-tau), where abnormal phosphorylation of tau protein is linked to the progression of Alzheimer's disease. CSF analysis provides valuable insights into the underlying disease processes, aiding in early diagnosis and potentially allowing for interventions before significant cognitive decline occurs. Together, PET scans and CSF analyses represent potent tools in the fight against Alzheimer's disease, offering hope for earlier detection, better understanding of the disease mechanisms, and the development of targeted treatments.

These diagnostic tools empower healthcare professionals to identify at-risk individuals, monitor disease progression, and potentially intervene before symptoms impact daily life. Early detection opens doors to personalized care and research into disease-modifying therapies.

Importance of Early Detection in Preclinical Alzheimer's Disease

The importance of early detection in preclinical Alzheimer's disease cannot be overstated, as it significantly influences the potential to shape the trajectory of the disease. Here's a closer look at why early detection matters:

Timely Intervention: Detecting Alzheimer's in its preclinical phase allows individuals and healthcare providers to take proactive measures. Early intervention can slow the disease's progression, leading to an enhanced quality of life. During this crucial time, individuals can explore and implement lifestyle modifications, engage in cognitive exercises, and adopt various strategies to preserve cognitive function. These proactive steps can significantly change the course of the disease.

Strategies to Delay Onset: With early detection, individuals can implement targeted strategies to delay the onset of symptomatic Alzheimer's. Activities stimulating the brain, such as engaging in puzzles, learning new skills, maintaining social connections, and adhering to a diet supporting brain health, can all contribute to this effort. These measures can potentially extend the period of cognitive health and delay the emergence of Alzheimer's symptoms.

Support and Counseling: The knowledge that one is at risk of developing Alzheimer's can be emotionally challenging. Healthcare professionals are crucial in offering emotional support and guidance to individuals navigating this uncertainty. Counseling and support services help those at risk and their families, providing them with tools to cope with the knowledge of impending cognitive changes and the associated challenges.

Access to Clinical Trials: Early detection opens the door to participation in clinical trials for emerging treatments. These trials are vital for the development of disease-modifying therapies that could alter the course of Alzheimer's. Participation in clinical trials contributes to scientific advancements and offers potential benefits to individual participants through access to cutting-edge treatments.

In summary, identifying cases of preclinical Alzheimer's empowers individuals, caregivers, and healthcare providers to take a proactive stance toward the disease. It facilitates a strategic approach to managing the condition, aiming to delay progression and improve outcomes. Early detection is a critical step in the fight against Alzheimer's, offering hope for better management of this complex neurological condition and, ultimately, for finding effective treatments.

Stage 2: Mild Cognitive Impairment (MCI) Due to Alzheimer's Disease

As autumn faded into the chill of winter, the whispers of change grew into murmurs, marking my father's transition into Stage 2 of Alzheimer's disease. This stage brought more pronounced challenges for him and us both as we navigated this new chapter with determination and hope.

The signs of progression were subtle at first, much like the season's first snowflakes, gentle but persistent. His moments of forgetfulness became more frequent, conversations looping in circles as stories and questions repeated themselves as familiar songs played in a loop. In these moments, watching the struggle behind his eyes, I felt a profound mix of sadness and admiration for the man who had always been my pillar of strength.

Our daily routines adapted to this new rhythm. The calendar that once hung on the fridge, marked with birthdays and appointments, now included daily tasks and reminders, each note penned with love and encouragement. We introduced new strategies to aid his memory, like keeping a diary where he could jot down thoughts, events, and feelings, turning the pages into a tapestry of his experiences.

Communication took on new forms, a dance of patience and understanding. I learned to listen to his words and the emotions they carried, offering reassurance when frustration bubbled to the surface. Our conversations, once filled with debates and discussions, became softer, filled with reminiscences and reflections on the simple joys of life.

The physical manifestations of Stage 2 began to unfold, a gradual decline that required more hands-on assistance. Together, we modified the house, installing handrails and removing rugs to prevent falls. Each adjustment was a small fortress against the encroaching tide of Alzheimer's. I watched as he navigated these changes with a mixture of resilience and resignation, silently acknowledging the battles we were beginning to face.

Despite the challenges, we found new ways to connect and share moments of joy. Music became a bridge between us, the melodies and rhythms sparking memories and emotions. We spent afternoons listening to his favorite albums, each song unlocking doors to the past and bringing forth smiles and laughter that lit up the room.

As his daughter, I took on the role of caregiver, advocate, and companion, a trinity of responsibilities that I carried with pride and devotion. This role demanded much but gave back in ways I could never have anticipated. In caring for my father, I discovered depths of strength within myself, fueled by love and the bond we shared.

The journey through Stage 2 Alzheimer's was a testament to the power of adaptation, the importance of compassion, and the value of cherishing every moment. We faced each day with realism and optimism, acknowledging the difficulties while finding beauty amid struggles.

As the seasons turned, signaling the approach of another spring, we stood together amidst the challenges, a testament to the enduring spirit of family and the unyielding power of love. Our story, marked by the stages of Alzheimer's, was not defined by the losses but by the moments of connection, understanding, and unwavering support that guided us through the shadows and into the light of shared human experience.

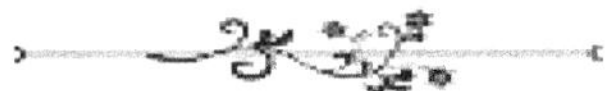

This phase marks a critical juncture in the progression of Alzheimer's disease, characterized by subtle yet significant cognitive changes that signal the onset of mild cognitive impairment (MCI), a precursor to Alzheimer's.

End-of-Life Planning: Discussions about end-of-life care and preferences become necessary. Though challenging, these conversations are essential to ensure that care aligns with the individual's and family's wishes.

Engage in advance care planning discussions with healthcare providers, the individual, and family members to make informed decisions about future care preferences and directives.

Legal and Financial Affairs: Ensuring that all legal documents are current and reflective of your loved one's wishes is paramount. This includes up-to-date wills, advance directives, and durable powers of attorney for healthcare and financial decisions. These documents protect your loved one's interests and honor their preferences. Consulting with an attorney specializing in elder law can provide guidance tailored to your situation. Additionally, meeting with a financial planner experienced in elder care planning can help navigate the complexities of financing long-term care, managing assets, and understanding potential benefits and entitlements.

Cognitive Changes Unveiled: During this stage, individuals may start experiencing mild memory lapses, such as misplacing everyday items or missing appointments, which become more frequent and noticeable. Finding words might be difficult, and recalling specific words or names during conversations poses a subtle challenge. Additionally, while still capable of managing independent daily activities, individuals may encounter mild difficulties in problem-solving and decision-making tasks.

Navigating the Gray Zone: These cognitive changes remain mild and do not significantly disrupt daily functioning. However, they act as early indicators of the more pronounced cognitive decline associated with Alzheimer's disease. This stage can be likened to a delicate balance, a tightrope walk between normalcy and the impending challenges of cognitive decline.

Noticeable Yet Tolerable: The changes are like a soft breeze at this stage—noticeable but not disruptive. Those close to the affected individual might observe these changes, such as the occasional memory lapse or the word that's just out of reach, but life continues relatively unchanged. Independence remains intact, albeit with subtle nuances that hint at the underlying condition.

The Race Against Alzheimer's: Early intervention is not just about delaying the progression of the disease; it's about preventing it. By catching MCI early, there's a potential to alter its course, delaying or even preventing the progression to full-blown Alzheimer's. It's a race against time, where knowledge is our ally and proactive action is our compass.

In navigating the delicate dance between cognition and change, embracing awareness and compassion and pursuing a brighter path forward is essential. The journey through MCI and potential progression to Alzheimer's underscores the importance of early detection, proactive lifestyle changes, and the collective effort to support those affected by this condition.

How Alzheimer's Disease is Diagnosed

Diagnosing Alzheimer's disease is a comprehensive process that aims to accurately assess and identify the presence of Alzheimer's disease while also ruling out other possible causes of dementia and cognitive decline. This multifaceted approach ensures the diagnosis is as accurate as possible, allowing for appropriate management and care planning. Below is a detailed overview of the diagnostic process for Alzheimer's disease.

Review of Medical History: The first step in diagnosing Alzheimer's is a detailed review of the patient's medical history. This includes discussing the patient's symptoms, their onset, and how they have progressed. The healthcare provider will also inquire about the patient's past medical issues, current health conditions, medications, and family history of neurological diseases to gather clues that might indicate the cause of cognitive changes.

Physical Examination: A physical examination helps to rule out other conditions that might be causing or contributing to the patient's symptoms. This examination may include checks for heart health, blood pressure, and other indicators of physical conditions that could affect cognitive functioning.

Neurological Assessment: Neurological examinations assess the functioning of the nervous system and can help identify signs of brain disorders other than Alzheimer's disease. These assessments may test reflexes, muscle strength, muscle tone, sense of touch and sight, coordination, and balance.

Cognitive and Memory Tests (Neuropsychological Testing): Cognitive testing is crucial for evaluating the patient's mental functions, including memory, language, problem-solving abilities, attention, and other aspects of cognitive health. Neuropsychological tests offer a detailed assessment of the patient's cognitive abilities and can help distinguish Alzheimer's disease from other types of dementia.

Brain Imaging Tests: Brain imaging technologies are used to visualize the structure and function of the brain, helping to rule out other causes of dementia-like symptoms, such as strokes, tumors, or fluid buildup. Standard imaging tests include:

Magnetic Resonance Imaging (MRI): MRI scans provide detailed images of the brain's structure, helping to identify shrinkage in specific areas affected by Alzheimer's disease, such as the hippocampus.

Computed Tomography (CT) Scans: CT scans can quickly provide brain images and help rule out brain tumors, strokes, or brain structure problems.

Positron Emission Tomography (PET) Scans: PET scans can detect brain plaques commonly associated with Alzheimer's disease. In some cases, PET scans can assess brain metabolism and function, offering insights into how well different brain regions are working.

Biomarker Tests: Advancements in Alzheimer's research have led to the development of biomarker tests that can detect changes in the brain and body fluids associated with Alzheimer's disease. These tests may measure levels of beta-amyloid and tau proteins in the cerebrospinal fluid or use specialized PET imaging techniques to detect amyloid plaques or tau tangles in the brain. However, these tests are typically used in research settings and may not be widely available in clinical practice.

Autopsy: A definitive diagnosis of Alzheimer's disease can only be made by examining brain tissue after death. Autopsies can reveal the presence of amyloid plaques and tau tangles, the hallmark pathological features of Alzheimer's disease.

The diagnostic process for Alzheimer's disease is thorough and multidisciplinary, involving a combination of clinical evaluations, cognitive testing, and imaging studies. Although a definitive diagnosis can be challenging to make during a patient's lifetime, these diagnostic tools allow healthcare providers to make a highly accurate presumptive diagnosis of Alzheimer's disease, facilitating early intervention and appropriate care planning.

Stage 3: Mild Alzheimer's Disease

Several years passed, and as the tender shoots of spring pushed through the thawing earth, signaling new beginnings, our family's journey with Alzheimer's disease transitioned into Stage 3. This stage brought more pronounced cognitive decline and increased care needs for my father. Yet, amidst these challenges, a new and unexpected dynamic unfolded within our home, offering glimpses of light in the shadow of Alzheimer's.

During the day, I had the joy and responsibility of caring for my grandson, Alex. A lively and curious soul, Alex became a constant presence in my father's world, their days intertwined like the threads of a well-loved quilt. This intergenerational bond, formed in the crucible of caregiving, brought forth moments of pure joy and poignant reminders of the cycle of life.

In Stage 3, my father's ability to engage in complex conversations diminished, and his memory lapses grew more profound. Yet, when Alex was by his side, a remarkable transformation occurred. The innocence and simplicity of a child's perspective seemed to bypass the barriers Alzheimer's had erected. Together, they shared activities that transcended the need for words—puzzles that challenged yet amused, coloring books that brought a riot of color to cloudy days and walks in the garden where my father could still name every flower, a remnant of a passion deeply ingrained.

Alex's presence brought a sense of normalcy and vitality to our home. His laughter filled the spaces that Alzheimer's sought to silence. In turn, despite the fog of confusion that often clouded his eyes, my father showed moments of lucidity and engagement that were becoming increasingly rare. It was as if Alex's youthful energy and unbridled enthusiasm breathed life into the embers of my father's fading memories.

The challenges of Stage 3 were ever-present. The need for assistance with daily activities became more pronounced, and safety concerns grew. We adapted our home further, ensuring my father and Alex a secure environment. I balanced my time between providing hands-on care for my father and nurturing my grandson, which was exhausting and incredibly rewarding.

In this stage, communication requires patience and creativity. With his innate adaptability, Alex learned to communicate with his great-grandfather in touching and ingenious ways. He would use simple words, gestures, and even drawings to convey his thoughts and feelings, often eliciting responses from my father that words alone could not.

As I observed their interactions, I realized Alex was learning valuable lessons about empathy, compassion, and the richness of human connection, even in the face of adversity. My father, despite the encroaching shadows of Alzheimer's, found a sense of purpose and joy in his relationship with Alex, a beacon of light in the twilight of his journey.

This period of our journey was a poignant reminder of life's cycles—of childhood's innocence intersecting with the wisdom of old age, each providing comfort and strength to the other. It reinforced the power of family, love, and the indomitable human spirit to find beauty and meaning, even as we navigated the complexities of Stage 3 Alzheimer's.

As the seasons changed, so too did our family's story, weaving a tapestry of memories that would endure, a testament to the enduring bonds of love that connected us all, from the youngest to the eldest, through the challenges and joys of life's journey.

In Stage 3 of Alzheimer's disease, known as Mild Alzheimer's Disease, symptoms become more evident and impactful.

Key Features

Cognitive Decline: In Stage 3 of Alzheimer's disease, the cognitive decline becomes more pronounced, affecting various aspects of daily functioning. Individuals with Mild Alzheimer's Disease may struggle with memory loss, including forgetting recent events or conversations. Language difficulties, such as finding the right words or following conversations, may arise. Reasoning and problem-solving abilities also deteriorate, making managing finances or planning more challenging.

These cognitive changes often lead to increased confusion and disorientation. Individuals may struggle remembering familiar places or faces and require more assistance with daily activities. While Mild Alzheimer's Disease marks a significant progression in the condition, individuals at this stage can still maintain some independence with support from caregivers and appropriate interventions.

Functional Impairment: Functional impairment in individuals with cognitive decline manifests in various ways, significantly impacting their ability to perform daily tasks. As the condition progresses, challenges become more apparent, particularly in managing finances, planning, and organizing activities. Here's an in-depth exploration of functional impairment:

Managing Finances: Individuals may need help paying bills, balancing checkbooks, or understanding financial statements. These difficulties arise from impaired mathematical skills and memory deficits, leading to errors, missed payments, and financial mismanagement.

Planning and Organizing: Planning activities, events, or daily routines become challenging. People may forget appointments, neglect essential tasks, or find it hard to follow schedules. Their organizational skills must improve, leading to cluttered spaces and difficulty prioritizing.

Decline in Cognitive Abilities: Functional impairment is closely tied to the progressive decline in cognitive functions such as memory, language, reasoning, and problem-solving. These cognitive deficits exacerbate the challenges in managing finances, planning, and organizing as individuals struggle to comprehend, remember, and execute tasks effectively.

In summary, functional impairment represents a significant hurdle for individuals with cognitive decline, affecting their independence and quality of life. Caregivers play a crucial role in providing support and assistance tailored to the specific needs of individuals at each stage of the disease. Caregiving for someone with Stage 3 Alzheimer's disease involves navigating a complex landscape of cognitive decline while striving to preserve the individual's dignity, independence, and quality of life. This stage, characterized by moderate to severe cognitive impairment, presents unique challenges and demands an adaptive, compassionate caregiving approach. Below, we elaborate on the caregiving strategies for Stage 3 Alzheimer's, offering deeper insights and additional tips to support caregivers in their vital role.

Assist with Daily Activities: As cognitive and physical abilities continue to decline in Stage 3, assistance with activities of daily living (ADLs) becomes increasingly critical. Caregivers should adopt a patient, supportive approach, allowing the individual to perform tasks to the best of their ability to maintain a sense of autonomy. When offering help, it's beneficial to use step-by-step instructions and provide hands-on assistance only when necessary. Encouraging the use of adaptive equipment can also promote independence in activities such as eating and dressing.

Maintain Routine: A consistent daily routine offers structure and predictability, comforting for someone with Stage 3 Alzheimer's. When establishing routines, consider the individual's lifelong habits and preferences to make the daily schedule as familiar and reassuring as possible. Incorporate regular times for meals, personal care, activities, and rest. A visual schedule can be helpful, using pictures or simple phrases to outline the day's plan, aiding comprehension and reducing anxiety.

Encourage Engagement: Tailor activities to the person's interests, abilities, and history. For instance, someone who enjoys gardening might enjoy tending to indoor plants or looking through gardening magazines. Sensory activities like listening to music, hand massage, or aromatherapy can provide comfort and stimulation. Reminiscence therapy, involving sharing memories from the past, can be advantageous and an opportunity to connect personally.

Ensure Safety: Modifications to the living environment are essential to prevent accidents and ensure safety. Conduct a thorough home safety assessment to identify potential hazards, such as loose rugs, poor lighting, and cluttered walkways, and make necessary adjustments. Consider using assistive technologies like motion sensors, video monitoring, and emergency call systems to enhance safety. Assess the individual's ability to safely use appliances and tools and make necessary adaptations or restrictions.

Effective Communication: Communication challenges in Stage 3 Alzheimer's require caregivers to adopt strategies that facilitate understanding and connection. Use short, simple sentences and avoid open-ended questions that can be overwhelming. Instead, offer choices between two options when possible. Nonverbal cues like gestures and facial expressions can also aid communication. Always approach from the front to avoid startling, and ensure you have the person's attention before speaking.

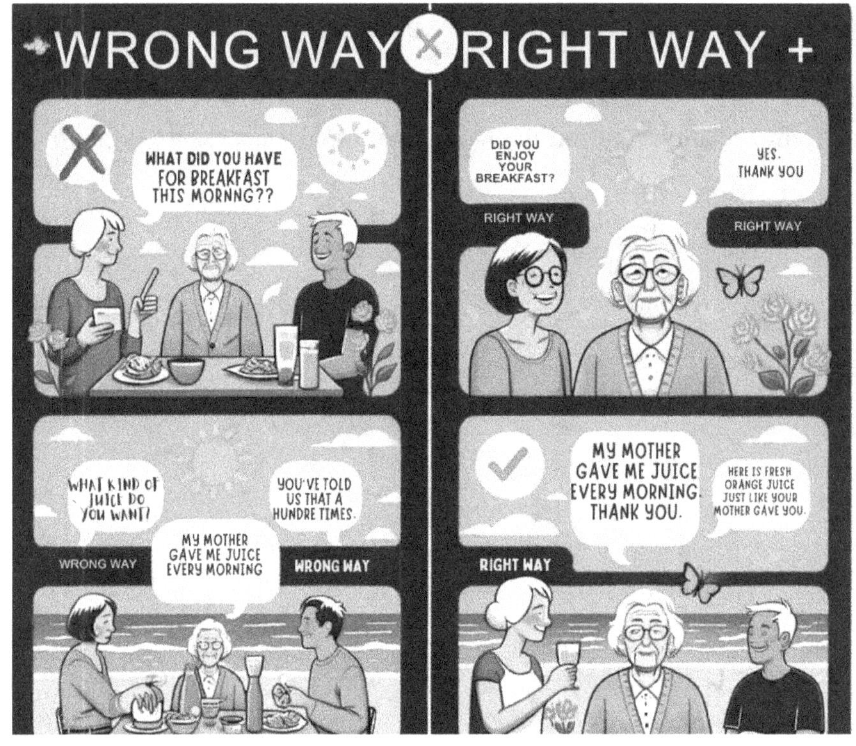

Provide Emotional Support: Emotional well-being is as important as physical health for someone with Alzheimer's. Listen actively, showing empathy and validation for their feelings. It's common for individuals in Stage 3 to experience frustration, sadness, or anger; acknowledging these emotions without judgment can provide significant comfort. Physical contact, like holding hands or a gentle touch, can convey support and reassurance when words may not suffice.

Build a Support Network: Caring for someone with Stage 3 Alzheimer's is a demanding task that can take a toll on the caregiver's health and well-being. Building a support network, including family, friends, and professional caregivers, can provide respite and support. Joining a caregiver support group in person or online can offer valuable advice, resources, and emotional support.

Seek Professional Guidance: Regular consultations with healthcare professionals specializing in Alzheimer's care can help manage symptoms, make caregiving decisions, and plan for the future. These professionals can offer insights into palliative care options, medication management, and strategies for effectively handling behavioral challenges.

By adopting a comprehensive, compassionate approach to caregiving, incorporating these strategies, and seeking support when needed, caregivers can significantly impact the lives of individuals with Stage 3 Alzheimer's, helping them navigate this stage with dignity and a sense of being cared for and valued.

Stage 4: Moderate Alzheimer's Disease

Four years had woven their passage through the fabric of our lives, each thread a testament to resilience, love, and the relentless march of time. As we navigated into Stage 4 of Alzheimer's with my father, the landscape of our daily existence had transformed significantly, reflecting the profound shifts not only in his condition but in the dynamics of our family life. Alex, now older, carried with him the lessons and memories of his early childhood spent in his great-grandfather's company, a bond forged in the simplicity and depth of shared moments.

Stage 4 ushered in more severe cognitive decline, and with it, the necessity for constant care became our new reality. My father, once a beacon of stories and wisdom, now was adrift in a sea of confusion, his clarity moments fading like the sun's last rays at dusk. The conversations we once shared had become rare jewels, treasured and poignant in their scarcity.

Alex, now stepping into the stride of his journey, became a young guardian of sorts, his understanding and empathy shaped by the years of loving and knowing his great-grandfather through the lens of Alzheimer's. Though less frequent due to the demands of school and growing independence, his visits remained a source of joy for my father, stirring the embers of recognition and happiness.

The progression of Alzheimer's demands adaptations and adjustments in every aspect of care. The house, already modified in previous stages, became a sanctuary designed to meet the evolving needs of my father's condition. Safety measures were intensified, and routines were meticulously planned and executed to provide structure and familiarity in a world that seemed increasingly foreign to him.

In this stage, our caregiving strategies evolved. The focus shifted towards preserving dignity, managing medical complexities, and providing comfort. We enlisted the help of home health aides to assist with the physical aspects of care, ensuring my father's needs were met with compassion and professionalism. Medical appointments became more frequent, a testament to the vigilance required to monitor his health and address the myriad challenges that accompanied his decline.

Yet, amidst the challenges, there were moments of unexpected grace. On good days, my father would join Alex and me in the garden, a place that had always been a source of solace for him. We would guide his hands to feel the textures of the plants, breathe in the scents of the flowers, and bask in the sun's warmth. In these moments, there was a sense of peace, a fleeting return to the essence of who my father had always been—a man deeply connected to the natural world.

Alex, with the intuition of the young and the wisdom gained from his unique relationship with his great-grandfather, often found ways to connect. He would bring drawings and school projects, sharing his world with a patience and tenderness that belied his years. In turn, my father, even in his diminished state, responded with smiles and laughter, a silent affirmation of the bond that remained unbroken by the ravages of Alzheimer's.

Navigating Stage 4 was a journey of love, loss, and the poignant beauty of caregiving. It was a testament to the strength of family ties, the resilience of the human spirit, and the profound impact of intergenerational relationships. As we moved forward, each day brought its challenges and rewards, reminding us of the preciousness of time and the enduring power of love.

As the years continued their relentless march, we faced the future with a blend of hope and realism, fortified by the memories of the past and the presence of love that transcended the boundaries of memory and time. In the heart of our family, my father's legacy lived on, not just in the stories we would tell but in the lessons of compassion, resilience, and unconditional love that would guide us through the coming days.

Stage 4 of Alzheimer's disease, often categorized as moderate Alzheimer's, signifies a crucial juncture in the progression of the condition. The cognitive decline and functional impairments that define this stage present significant challenges to the individuals experiencing them and their caregivers. The deepening memory loss, communication difficulties, and challenges in daily activities necessitate a comprehensive, compassionate approach to care. Here, we explore the complexities of Stage 4 Alzheimer's in more detail, offering enhanced insights and caregiving strategies to support those navigating this difficult phase.

Understanding Severe Cognitive Decline: In Stage 4 Alzheimer's, the cognitive faculties of affected individuals deteriorate noticeably. Memory loss extends beyond simple forgetfulness to a pronounced inability to recall critical personal information, significant events or even recognize close family members and friends. This severe cognitive decline disrupts daily life, affecting not only memory but also the ability to perform tasks, understand information, and engage in social activities.

Challenges in Communication: Communication becomes increasingly challenging as individuals may struggle to find words, follow along with conversations, or express their thoughts and needs effectively. This can lead to frustration and isolation, both for the person with Alzheimer's and their caregivers. Understanding and patience become key in facilitating communication and ensuring that the individual feels heard and supported.

Functional Impairment: The impairments in cognitive functions translate into difficulties with daily living activities. Individuals may require assistance with personal care, including hygiene, dressing, eating, and mobility. The loss of independence can be distressing, emphasizing the need for sensitive support that respects the individual's dignity.

Caregiving Strategies for Severe Cognitive Decline

Enhancing Recognition: Photographs and Personal Items: Utilize photographs of family members, friends, and significant life events as memory aids. Labeling these photos can help individuals recall names and relationships, facilitating a connection to their past. Personal items that hold sentimental value can also act as powerful triggers for reminiscence, aiding in maintaining a connection with the individual's history and identity.

Facilitating Communication

Simplify Language: Use simple, straightforward sentences and avoid complex or abstract concepts that might confuse the individual.

When giving instructions, break them down into manageable, step-by-step processes to make tasks more achievable.

Repetition and Patience: Be prepared to repeat information and instructions multiple times. It's essential to display patience and understanding, recognizing that the individual's capacity to process and retain information is significantly impaired.

Nonverbal Communication: Embrace nonverbal cues, including gestures, facial expressions, and touch, to support and enhance verbal communication. These nonverbal forms can convey meaning and emotion, helping to bridge gaps where verbal communication may fall short.

Adopting these caregiving strategies can help address the challenges of severe cognitive decline. By enhancing recognition and facilitating communication, caregivers can support the individual's sense of self, promote understanding, and foster a positive, nurturing environment. It's also essential for caregivers to seek support for themselves, ensuring they have the resources and resilience needed to provide compassionate care.

Creating a Supportive Environment

Creating a supportive environment and addressing functional impairments are critical components of caregiving for individuals experiencing severe cognitive decline, such as those with Stage 4 Alzheimer's. Here's how caregivers can implement these strategies effectively:

Safe, Calm Spaces: Minimizing environmental stressors by maintaining a calm and quiet living space is essential. Removing clutter and potential hazards can prevent falls and injuries. Implementing safety measures such as locks and alarms can prevent wandering and ensure the individual's safety within their environment.

Addressing Functional Impairments

Adaptive Devices and Aids: Adaptive clothing, eating utensils, and other aids can facilitate independence in daily activities. For example, wearing Velcro closures and non-slip socks can enhance comfort and safety, making personal care tasks easier and safer for the individual.

Personal Care Assistance: It is crucial to provide personal care with sensitivity and respect for the individual's privacy and autonomy. Encouraging participation in self-care to the extent possible while offering assistance as needed helps maintain the individual's dignity.

Emotional and Social Support

Encourage Social Interaction: Maintaining social connections is vital for the emotional well-being of individuals with Alzheimer's. Facilitating visits with family and friends and adapting social activities to the individual's abilities can foster enjoyment and engagement.

Emotional Reassurance: Providing constant emotional support and reassurance is key. Affirming the individual's feelings and experiences offers comfort and understanding, helping them navigate the emotional challenges of the disease.

Navigating the care of someone with Stage 4 Alzheimer's involves a comprehensive approach that combines practical care strategies with emotional and social support. Understanding the unique challenges and adapting caregiving approaches allows caregivers to provide compassionate and practical support. This approach not only addresses the complex needs of those affected by Alzheimer's but also honors their dignity and individuality, enhancing their quality of life as the disease progresses.

Functional Impairment

The decline in cognitive abilities significantly affects the capability to perform basic ADLs. Individuals in Stage 4 will need considerable assistance with personal care tasks, including dressing, bathing, and toileting.

Caregiving Strategies: Establish a routine for personal care tasks, performing them in the same order and at the same time each day to create a sense of familiarity and security.

Enhance bathroom safety with grab bars, raised toilet seats, and non-slip mats. Consider supervised bathing for safety.

Behavioral and Psychological Symptoms: Behavioral and psychological symptoms of dementia (BPSD) become more prominent in Stage 4. Agitation, aggression, wandering, and sundowning are common.

Sundowning, also known as "late-day confusion," is a symptom that commonly affects individuals with Alzheimer's disease. It refers to the increased confusion, agitation, anxiety, and restlessness that typically occurs in the late afternoon, evening, or night. While the exact cause of sundowning is not fully understood, it is believed to be related to changes in the brain that affect an individual's internal body clock, leading to disruptions in the sleep-wake cycle. Environmental factors, such as reduced lighting and increased shadows, can also contribute to the symptoms of sundowning. Strategies to manage sundowning include maintaining a routine, increasing lighting in the evening, and providing calming activities to reduce agitation.

Implement structured daily activities that provide a sense of purpose and reduce boredom, which can trigger behavioral issues. Create a safe, wander-proof environment. Use door alarms and GPS devices to monitor and ensure safety. Approach behavioral challenges with empathy, trying to identify the underlying cause, such as discomfort, pain, or unmet needs. Distraction and redirection can be effective in managing agitation or aggression. Maintain a tranquil environment, especially in the evening, to help mitigate sundowning. Avoid overstimulation.

Communication Challenges: As cognitive decline progresses, communication becomes increasingly difficult. Individuals may need help finding words, forming coherent sentences, or understanding complex instructions. Encourage nonverbal communication through gestures, facial expressions, and touch to convey meaning and comfort. Simplify conversations, using yes-or-no questions or offering choices between two options to facilitate decision-making. Listen attentively and offer reassurance, validating feelings even when verbal communication is limited.

Support for Caregivers: The increasing demands of caregiving at this stage can lead to caregiver burnout. Caregivers must seek support through family, professional caregivers, or support groups. Explore respite care options to provide temporary relief from caregiving duties, allowing time for rest and self-care. Engage with caregiver support groups and Alzheimer's associations for resources, education, and emotional support. Consider consulting with healthcare providers for guidance on managing specific challenges and planning for the progression of the disease.

Navigating Stage 4 of Alzheimer's disease requires a multifaceted approach that balances the individual's needs with the caregiver's well-being. By adapting caregiving strategies to address the unique challenges of this stage, caregivers can provide compassionate care that maintains their loved one's dignity and comfort.

Stage 5: Late-Stage Alzheimer's

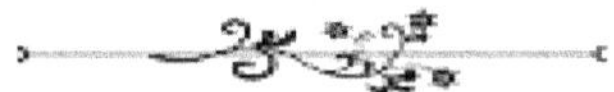

As we journeyed into Stage 5, the final stage of Alzheimer's, the fabric of our family story was threaded with both the deepest shades of challenge and the lightest hues of love's enduring presence. My father's decline into severe cognitive and physical impairment necessitated decisions that weighed heavily on our hearts, leading to the transition into a specialized memory care facility. This decision, though fraught with sorrow and guilt, was made with love and the understanding that it was in his best interest, ensuring he received the constant, professional care his condition now demanded.

The memory care facility was a place of warmth and compassion, designed to provide a haven for individuals like my father. The staff were angels in disguise, offering medical care and a sense of community and dignity for those in the twilight of their lives. Despite the reassurance that my father was in good hands, the emotional toll of seeing him in this new environment, further removed from the man he once was, struck chords of grief and longing for days gone by.

Alex, now coming into his own, had grown up with the shadow of Alzheimer's ever-present. His relationship with his great-grandfather had shaped him profoundly and subtly, imbuing him with an empathy and depth that few his age possessed. However, as Stage 5 progressed, Alex decided to halt his visits. He wanted to preserve the memory of his great-grandfather as the loving, gentle soul he knew in his heart rather than witness the final, most challenging phase of the disease. This decision, though painful, was met with understanding and respect. Alex's love for his great-grandfather remained untarnished, a beacon of their shared past.

The day my father passed away was quiet, a stark contrast to the storm of emotions raging within me. I sat by his side, holding his hand, a silent witness to the final moments of his journey. The room was filled with a profound sense of peace, as if my father, too, understood that it was time to let go. In those last breaths, I whispered words of love and gratitude, thanking him for the lessons he taught me, for the strength he instilled, and for the unconditional love he gave freely, even in the face of Alzheimer's relentless march.

His passing was a moment of poignant release, a mixture of profound loss and the relief that his struggle had come to an end. In the days that followed, as we gathered to honor his life, the legacy of his love and the strength of our family bonds were palpable. Although Alex chose not to be present in the final moments, he shared his tribute, a heartfelt testament to his great-grandfather's impact on his life, a reminder that love's influence transcends physical presence.

As we navigated the aftermath of my father's passing, the journey through Alzheimer's remained a testament to the power of memory, the resilience of the human spirit, and the indelible impact of love. Bound by our shared experience, Alex and I continued to honor my father's memory in our daily lives, cherishing the moments we had and the lessons we learned.

In the end, our story was not defined by the sorrow of Alzheimer's but by the strength it revealed within us, the depth of our connections, and the enduring legacy of love that my father left behind. His journey through Alzheimer's, though marked by loss, was also a journey of discovery, revealing the unbreakable bonds of family and the transcendent power of love to guide us through life's most challenging moments.

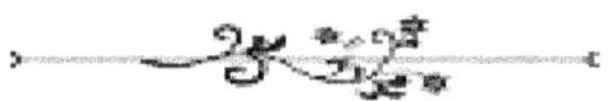

In the final stage of Alzheimer's disease, also known as severe or late-stage Alzheimer's, individuals undergo profound cognitive and functional impairment. This stage demands intensive caregiving efforts focused on comfort, dignity, and quality of life as individuals lose their independence and face significant health challenges. Caregiving strategies must be adapted to address the complex needs of those with Stage 5 Alzheimer's, emphasizing compassionate care and symptom management. Here, we expand on the caregiving strategies for Stage 5 Alzheimer's. Here is guidance for caregivers navigating this demanding phase:

Assist with Activities of Daily Living (ADLs): In Stage 5, individuals require comprehensive assistance with all ADLs, as they may no longer perform these tasks independently due to cognitive and physical decline.

- **Caregiving Strategies**: Establish a gentle, patient approach to personal care, respecting the individual's privacy and dignity. Use encouraging words and simple, step-by-step instructions to guide them through each activity.
- Adapt the environment and use assistive devices to simplify ADLs, such as using a shower chair for bathing or clothing with easy closures for dressing.

Manage Medical Needs: The risk of medical complications, including infections, malnutrition, and dehydration, increases significantly in this stage, necessitating vigilant care and coordination with healthcare providers.

- **Caregiving Strategies:** Maintain a strict medication management regimen, ensuring medications are administered correctly and on time to manage symptoms and prevent complications.
- Regularly communicate with healthcare professionals to monitor the individual's health status, adjusting care plans based on their guidance.

Create a Calm and Safe Environment: As cognitive decline deepens, individuals may become more prone to anxiety, agitation, and wandering, making a safe, calm environment crucial.

- **Caregiving Strategies:** Implement safety measures such as installing bed rails, using door alarms, and removing hazards to prevent falls and ensure the individual's safety.

- Use soothing techniques, such as soft music, gentle touch, and maintaining a quiet environment, to help manage agitation and promote a sense of calm.

Encourage Social Engagement and Meaningful Activities: Maintaining social connections and engaging in meaningful activities can enhance the quality of life, even as communication and cognitive abilities decline.

- **Caregiving Strategies:** Facilitate visits from family and friends, encouraging them to interact through touch, music, or simply being present, which can provide comfort and stimulation.

- Introduce sensory stimulation activities tailored to the individual's preferences and abilities, such as listening to their favorite music, and tactile activities like holding soft fabrics or aromatherapy.

Provide Emotional Support: Emotional support becomes paramount in Stage 5, as individuals may experience distress or discomfort without effectively communicating their needs.

- **Caregiving Strategies:** Show empathy and patience, reassuring through words, touch, and presence to convey love and care.

- Recognize and respond to nonverbal cues of discomfort or distress, such as facial expressions or body language, to address needs promptly.

- Seek support from palliative care services, which can provide comprehensive symptom management and emotional support for both the individual and caregivers during this stage.

Caregiving in Stage 5 Alzheimer's demands a holistic approach that balances medical care with emotional support, safety, and dignity. By implementing these strategies, caregivers can provide compassionate care that addresses the complex needs of their loved ones, ensuring their final stage of life is as comfortable and meaningful as possible.

Treatment of Alzheimer's Disease

Current Treatments for Alzheimer's Disease

While there is no cure for Alzheimer's disease, there are treatments available that can help manage symptoms for some patients. Current treatments include:

Medications for Cognitive Symptoms: Cholinesterase inhibitors (e.g., donepezil, rivastigmine, and galantamine) and memantine are prescribed to manage memory loss, confusion, and problems with thinking and reasoning.

Medications for Behavioral and Psychiatric Symptoms: These include antidepressants, antipsychotic medications, and anxiolytics to manage depression, aggression, and agitation.

Supportive Therapies: Cognitive stimulation therapy, exercise, and activities can help maintain cognition and physical health.

Experimental Treatments for Alzheimer's Disease

Research into new treatments for Alzheimer's disease is ongoing and includes:

Amyloid and Tau Targeting Treatments: aim to reduce amyloid plaques or prevent tau tangles, which are hallmarks of Alzheimer's disease.

Immunotherapy involves using monoclonal antibodies to clear amyloid plaques from the brain.

Lifestyle Interventions: Research explores how diet, exercise, and cognitive training may influence the progression of Alzheimer's disease.

Gene Therapy: Experimental approaches are being studied to correct or compensate for genetic mutations that cause Alzheimer's.

Clinical trials are crucial for developing new treatments. Participation in these trials advances medical knowledge and offers patients access to the latest treatment innovations.

The landscape of Alzheimer's disease diagnosis and treatment is evolving, with ongoing research aimed at understanding the disease better and finding more effective ways to treat it. Families facing Alzheimer's are encouraged to seek comprehensive care that includes medical treatment, supportive therapies, and participation in clinical trials as appropriate.

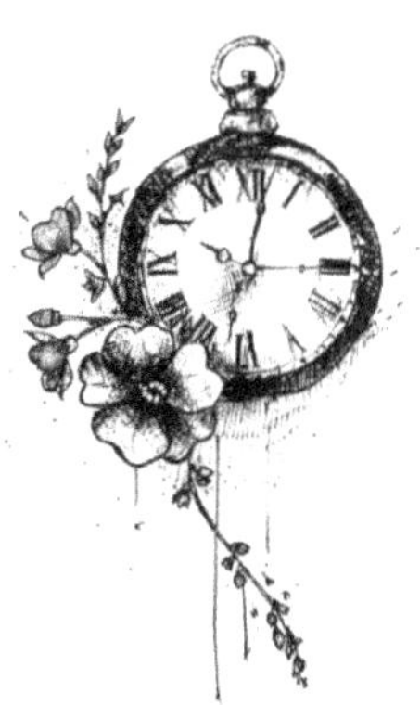

Chapter 2: Caring for Someone with Alzheimer's Disease

Understanding the Caregiver's Role

The caregiver's role in the journey of Alzheimer's disease cannot be overstated, embodying a beacon of support, empathy, and understanding for the individual navigating the uncertain waters of this condition. As Alzheimer's disease progresses, its impact deepens, not just on the cognitive and physical capabilities of the person affected but also on their emotional and psychological well-being. In this evolving landscape, the caregiver becomes an indispensable pillar, offering the support and assistance necessary for the person with Alzheimer's to maintain as much dignity and quality of life as possible.

The responsibilities that fall upon a caregiver's shoulders are varied and profound. They extend beyond managing medical appointments and administering medications, tasks that, while critical, barely scratch the surface of the caregiver's comprehensive role. Caregivers are intimately involved in assisting with the personal care of their loved ones, ensuring that hygiene, dressing, and nutrition are met with respect and sensitivity to preserve the individual's dignity.

Moreover, the caregiver's responsibility includes creating and maintaining a safe living environment. This involves adapting the home to meet the changing needs of the person with Alzheimer's, safeguarding against potential hazards that could lead to injury, and implementing strategies to manage risks such as wandering, which becomes more prevalent as the disease advances.

However, the role of a caregiver transcends these practical tasks, delving into the realms of emotional support and companionship. The psychological toll of Alzheimer's on individuals can manifest as feelings of confusion, frustration, and isolation. Caregivers serve as a constant source of comfort and stability, offering reassurance and understanding that helps mitigate these emotional challenges. Through their presence, caregivers provide a sense of normalcy and continuity, reminding the individual of their identity and worth beyond the disease.

The companionship offered by caregivers also plays a crucial role in maintaining the social engagement of the person with Alzheimer's. By facilitating interactions with friends and family, caregivers help sustain the social connections vital for emotional health and well-being. These interactions can spark joy and recognition, offering respite from the daily struggles with memory and cognition.

The caregiver's role is multifaceted, encompassing the physical, emotional, and social support dimensions necessary for navigating Alzheimer's disease. It is a role marked by challenges, sacrifices, profound rewards, and deep bonds. Caregivers enhance the quality of life for those they care for and embody the resilience of the human spirit in the face of adversity. Their dedication and love provide the critical support that enables individuals with Alzheimer's to face each day with dignity and a sense of personal worth, making caregivers unsung heroes in the journey through Alzheimer's disease.

The Challenges of Being a Caregiver

The role of a caregiver for someone with Alzheimer's disease is imbued with challenges that extend far beyond the scope of ordinary daily tasks and responsibilities. The physical and emotional demands placed upon caregivers are immense, often pushing the boundaries of their endurance and resilience. At the heart of these challenges lies the stress and emotional turmoil that accompanies the journey of caring for a loved one undergoing the relentless progression of Alzheimer's.

One of the most profound struggles caregivers face is the emotional pain of witnessing the gradual decline of someone they deeply care about. This decline is not merely a loss of memory or cognitive function but a gradual fading of the person's identity and the shared memories that once defined their relationship. The emotional weight of this loss can evoke a complex tapestry of feelings, including grief for the progressive losses, frustration at the disease's unyielding nature, and guilt over feelings of inadequacy or moments of impatience.

Furthermore, the all-consuming nature of caregiving can lead to significant changes in the caregiver's social and personal life. The time and energy demands of caregiving—from managing medical appointments and daily care routines to addressing crises—can severely limit the caregiver's ability to maintain social connections, pursue personal interests, or even attend to their health and well-being. This isolation can exacerbate feelings of loneliness, stress, and depression, creating a difficult-to-break cycle.

The impact of caregiving on the caregiver's health is another critical concern. The chronic stress associated with caregiving duties can lead to physical health problems, including increased risks for chronic conditions such as hypertension, heart disease, and weakened immune function. Emotional health suffers as well, with caregivers exhibiting higher rates of anxiety, depression, and other mental health challenges.

Moreover, the demands of caregiving can also affect the caregiver's work life and financial stability. Balancing caregiving responsibilities with professional obligations can lead to reduced working hours, loss of income, or even job loss. The financial strain and the cost of care-related expenses can add stress and uncertainty to the caregiver's life.

Relationships with other family members can also be strained as the dynamics within the family shift in response to the caregiving situation. Disagreements over care decisions, financial contributions, and the distribution of caregiving tasks can lead to conflicts that further erode the caregiver's support network.

Despite these challenges, caregivers persist, driven by love, duty, and the deep human connection they share with their loved ones. Their journey is one of profound sacrifice and resilience, highlighting the need for greater support and recognition of the vital role they play in the lives of those with Alzheimer's disease. Acknowledging caregivers' challenges is the first step toward providing the support, resources, and understanding they need to navigate this complex path with strength and compassion.

The Rewards of Being a Caregiver

As the author of this book, I am honored to share a heartfelt story about the profound rewards of being a caregiver for my next-door neighbor in North Carolina. In our bustling neighborhood, filled with the warmth of community spirit, I was drawn to the quiet strength and unwavering kindness of Mrs. Johnson, a beloved member of our tight-knit enclave.

When Mrs. Johnson faced the challenges of aging and declining health, I embarked on a journey of compassion and caregiving that forever changed my perspective on life. Through the countless hours spent by her side, offering comfort, companionship, and support, I discovered the true meaning of empathy and selflessness.

Despite the trials and tribulations of caregiving, I found immeasurable joy in the simple moments I shared with Mrs. Johnson—from lively conversations over cups of tea to quiet walks in the neighborhood park. Each day brought new opportunities for connection and understanding, deepening our bond and enriching our lives in ways I never imagined possible.

Through the highs and lows of caregiving, I learned that the most significant rewards are often found in the smallest acts of kindness. Mrs. Johnson's smile of gratitude, the warmth of her embrace, and the profound sense of purpose that filled my heart were the true treasures of my journey as a caregiver.

In caring for Mrs. Johnson, I discovered the transformative power of compassion and the extraordinary capacity of the human spirit to uplift and inspire. And though our time together may have been fleeting, the memories we shared and the lessons we learned will forever remain etched in my heart.

This story is a testament to the profound rewards of being a caregiver – the bonds formed, the lives touched, and the enduring legacy of love and compassion that transcends time and space.

Despite the challenges, caregiving can be gratifying. Many caregivers find deep satisfaction in providing care and support, strengthening their bond with their loved ones. It can be fulfilling to know that you are making a significant difference in the quality of life of someone with Alzheimer's. Caregiving can also lead to personal growth as caregivers develop new skills, resilience, and a deeper appreciation for the value of each moment. The caregiving journey often brings unexpected moments of joy, tenderness, and closeness, offering a unique perspective on the meaning of love and the strength of the human spirit.

Understanding the caregiver's role is the first step in navigating the complex journey of Alzheimer's care. Acknowledging the challenges and the rewards is crucial in preparing oneself for the path ahead, ensuring that caregivers prioritize their well-being alongside that of their loved ones.

Providing Physical Care

Caring for someone with Alzheimer's disease involves a wide range of responsibilities, including the essential tasks of assisting with bathing, grooming, dressing, feeding, and managing incontinence. These aspects of care are vital for maintaining the dignity, comfort, and health of a person living with Alzheimer's.

Bathing and Grooming

As Alzheimer's disease progresses, the seemingly simple acts of bathing and grooming can evolve into complex challenges fraught with emotional and physical hurdles for both the individual with Alzheimer's and their caregiver. These personal care activities, intrinsic to our sense of dignity and self-esteem, can become sources of distress and confusion for someone whose cognitive abilities are declining. For caregivers, navigating these challenges requires empathy, patience, and practical strategies to ensure that bathing and grooming are conducted with respect and sensitivity to the individual's needs and emotions.

Maintaining a routine for bathing and grooming is paramount. The power of routine lies in its ability to instill a sense of predictability and security in an individual with Alzheimer's, who may find comfort in the familiarity of a structured sequence of activities. By establishing a consistent schedule for these personal care tasks, caregivers can help mitigate the confusion and anxiety that changes in routine may provoke. This consistency becomes a cornerstone of care, helping preserve the individual's sense of time and sequence, often eroded by the disease.

Ensuring privacy and warmth during bathing and grooming is another critical aspect of care. These moments are inherently personal and can make an individual feel particularly vulnerable, especially in the later stages of Alzheimer's, when understanding and communication may be significantly impaired. Caregivers must protect their loved one's dignity, cover them with towels or bathrobes when not actively bathing, and maintain a warm environment to prevent discomfort or distress.

The approach taken by the caregiver during these activities can significantly impact the individual's experience. A calm and reassuring voice helps to soothe anxieties and communicates care and respect. Explaining each step before proceeding allows the individual with Alzheimer's to anticipate what comes next, reducing potential surprises that could trigger agitation or resistance. This gentle guidance helps bridge the gap between the caregiver's intent to assist and the individual's need for autonomy.

Allowing the person with Alzheimer's to participate in their care as much as possible fosters a sense of independence and agency. Even if their participation is limited, encouraging them to engage in simple tasks, such as holding a washcloth or brushing their hair, can contribute to their sense of self-worth and involvement in their care. This empowerment is a delicate balance that respects the individual's abilities while providing the necessary support to ensure their safety and well-being.

Bathing and grooming in the context of Alzheimer's care are more than mere tasks; they allow caregivers to express their compassion, respect, and support for their loved one's dignity. By adopting a thoughtful, patient approach, caregivers can transform these challenging moments into experiences that reinforce the individual's sense of self and provide comfort in the disorientation that Alzheimer's often brings.

Dressing and Feeding

The progression of Alzheimer's disease brings with it a series of challenges that extend into the most essential aspects of daily life, such as dressing and feeding. These tasks, which many of us perform without a second thought, can become significant hurdles for those living with Alzheimer's. The disease's impact on motor skills, coordination, and decision-making capacity means that caregivers must approach these activities thoughtfully and adaptively to support the individual's dignity, independence, and nutritional well-being.

Dressing with Dignity and Ease: As Alzheimer's progresses, choosing what to wear and the physical process of dressing can become sources of frustration and confusion. Caregivers can alleviate these challenges by selecting comfortable, easy-to-wear clothes that minimize the complexity of dressing. Clothing with simple fastenings, elastic waistbands, and Velcro closures can significantly reduce the physical demands of dressing, promoting an individual's sense of autonomy.

Laying clothes in the order they should be put on is another strategy that can streamline the dressing process. This helps clarify the sequence of actions needed to dress and offers a visual cue to guide the individual through each step, fostering a sense of achievement and reducing potential stress.

Adapting Feeding for Nutritional Well-being: Nutritional care is critical to caring for someone with Alzheimer's. As the disease affects swallowing and the ability to use standard eating utensils, caregivers must adapt mealtime practices to ensure the individual receives a balanced, nutritious diet. This adaptation might include preparing softer foods that are easier to chew and swallow, serving smaller portions more frequently throughout the day to align with the individual's appetite and attention span, and ensuring that meals are appealing and varied to stimulate interest in eating.

Adaptive utensils designed for those with limited dexterity can also significantly improve the ease with which individuals with Alzheimer's can feed themselves. These utensils, which often feature easy-grip handles or weighted bases, can help compensate for the loss of fine motor skills, allowing the individual to maintain independence and dignity during meals.

The Role of the Caregiver in Dressing and Feeding: For caregivers, assisting with dressing and feeding requires a delicate balance between providing necessary support and preserving the individual's sense of independence. This involves the practical aspects of selecting appropriate clothing and preparing suitable meals and the emotional support that acknowledges the individual's frustrations and successes in these everyday activities.

In dressing and feeding, caregivers can encourage and celebrate the individual's abilities while gently assisting where needed. This supportive approach can transform these daily tasks from potential sources of conflict into moments of connection and affirmation, reinforcing the individual's sense of self and providing structured, nurturing routines that anchor their day.

Ultimately, navigating the challenges of dressing and feeding in Alzheimer's care is emblematic of the broader caregiving journey: one that demands adaptability, patience, and a deep commitment to enhancing the quality of life for those living with Alzheimer's. Through thoughtful strategies and compassionate support, caregivers play a pivotal role in ensuring that the most essential aspects of daily life are infused with dignity and respect.

Managing Incontinence

Incontinence, a prevalent issue in the later stages of Alzheimer's disease, presents a profound challenge that requires caregivers to navigate a delicate balance between providing necessary care and preserving the dignity of their loved ones. As Alzheimer's progresses, the loss of control over bladder and bowel functions can be distressing for the individual, often accompanied by feelings of embarrassment and a diminished sense of self-worth. For caregivers, managing incontinence demands practical solutions and a deep well of empathy, understanding, and respect for the individual's feelings and experiences.

Establishing a Routine: One of the most effective strategies for managing incontinence involves establishing a regular toileting schedule. By encouraging bathroom visits at consistent times throughout the day, caregivers can often prevent accidents before they happen. This proactive approach requires careful observation and timing, aligning with the individual's natural rhythms and cues to the best extent possible. Regularity in toileting can help reduce the unpredictability of incontinence and provide a framework of routine that is reassuring for both the caregiver and the person with Alzheimer's.

Recognizing the Signs: Attention to the signs indicating a need to use the bathroom is crucial. As verbal communication abilities decline, individuals with Alzheimer's may struggle to express their needs directly.

Caregivers must become adept at interpreting non-verbal cues, such as restlessness, facial expressions, or gestures that may signify discomfort or an urgent need to go to the bathroom. Responding quickly and gently to these signals can help prevent accidents and reduce the individual's anxiety related to incontinence.

Using Protective Garments: Protective garments, such as absorbent underwear or pads, can provide an added layer of security for individuals with Alzheimer's, helping to manage incontinence with dignity. Selecting products that are comfortable, discreet, and easy to change is essential, as is ensuring that the individual's skin is cared for properly to prevent irritation or infections. Protective garments should be introduced sensitively, emphasizing their role in maintaining cleanliness and comfort.

Preserving Dignity: It is vital to approach incontinence with sensitivity and understanding. Caregivers should always strive to preserve the individual's dignity, treating them with the same respect and consideration they desire for themselves. This includes maintaining privacy during toileting and changing, using a calm and reassuring tone, and avoiding any language or behavior that could be interpreted as judgmental or punitive.

Adapting to Changing Needs: Providing physical care for someone with Alzheimer's requires adapting to their changing needs and preferences. What works well at one stage of the disease may not be effective later on, necessitating continual reassessment and adjustment of care strategies. Flexibility, coupled with a commitment to empathy and respect, forms the foundation of effective caregiving for incontinence and other challenges posed by Alzheimer's disease.

By approaching the management of incontinence with patience, compassion, and a focus on dignity, caregivers can help their loved ones navigate this problematic aspect of Alzheimer's with a sense of normalcy and respect. In doing so, they reinforce the value of each individual's experience, affirming that dignity and care are paramount, even in challenging circumstances.

Providing Emotional Care

Caring for a person with Alzheimer's disease extends beyond physical needs, encompassing vital emotional support. Understanding and addressing the emotional well-being of both the person with Alzheimer's and the caregiver are crucial components of comprehensive care.

Communicating with Someone with Alzheimer's Disease

Communicating with someone who has Alzheimer's disease requires a thoughtful, patient approach that acknowledges the complexity of their experience. As the disease progresses, traditional conversation methods may no longer be effective, necessitating strategies beyond words to maintain a connection. Enhancing communication with someone with Alzheimer's facilitates better interaction and supports their dignity and well-being. Here's a deeper dive into practical communication techniques:

Speak Clearly and Simply: Alzheimer's can cause cognitive changes that challenge processing complex sentences. Speaking clearly and using simple, straightforward sentences can significantly improve understanding. When presenting choices, limiting options to avoid overwhelming them is helpful. For instance, rather than asking an open-ended question about what they'd like to eat, offering two specific choices can make it easier for them to decide and communicate their preference.

Maintain Eye Contact: Eye contact plays a crucial role in communication, serving as a nonverbal cue that signals engagement and sincerity. For individuals with Alzheimer's, maintaining eye contact during conversation can help hold their attention, making the interaction more meaningful. It reassures them they are being listened to and valued, fostering a sense of connection and personal respect.

Use Nonverbal Cues: As Alzheimer's progresses, the ability to understand and use language can decline, making nonverbal communication increasingly important. Body language, gestures, and tone of voice can convey information and emotions. Positive, encouraging gestures such as nodding, smiling, and gentle touches can offer comfort and reassurance, helping bridge verbal communication gaps. These cues can also assist in conveying the intent and emotion behind words, which may be particularly valuable when verbal comprehension is limited.

Listen with Patience: Listening is as crucial as speaking to effective communication. Offering the person with Alzheimer's ample time to respond without rushing them acknowledges their efforts to communicate and shows respect for their autonomy. It's essential to pay attention to their words and the emotions and intentions underlying their communication. Demonstrating patience and attempting to interpret their feelings and needs can lead to a deeper understanding and connection, even when their words may be unclear.

Additional Strategies

Redirect and Reassure: If the conversation becomes challenging or the individual becomes upset, gently redirecting the topic to something more comforting can be effective. Providing reassurance through calm, affirmative statements can help alleviate distress.

Engage in Reminiscing: People with Alzheimer's often retain long-term memories longer than short-term ones. Engaging in conversations about their past can be a meaningful way to connect and stimulate conversation, making them feel valued and heard.

Create a Positive Environment: Reducing background noise and distractions can help the individual focus on the conversation. A calm, quiet setting can enhance their ability to engage and respond.

Adopting these communication strategies requires empathy, flexibility, and a deep commitment to supporting the individual's dignity and quality of life. By tailoring interactions to meet their unique needs and abilities, caregivers can foster meaningful connections, reduce frustration, and enhance the well-being of individuals with Alzheimer's.

Managing Difficult Behaviors

Managing challenging behaviors in individuals with Alzheimer's disease demands a nuanced understanding of the disease's impact on cognition and emotion. As the disease progresses, it can lead to various challenging behaviors, including aggression, wandering, repeated questioning, or restlessness. These behaviors often express unmet needs, discomfort, or confusion rather than deliberate attempts to be complicated. Caregivers can employ various strategies to manage these behaviors effectively, always focusing on the individual's dignity and well-being.

Understanding the Cause: The first step in managing challenging behaviors is to look beyond the behavior and its underlying cause. Often, such behaviors are a response to something specific in the person's environment or a physical need that is not being met. For example, aggression might be triggered by physical discomfort, confusion, or fear, while wandering could respond to boredom or an unmet need for physical activity. Identifying triggers requires careful observation and sometimes a bit of detective work. Once the cause is understood, it becomes easier to address the root of the problem rather than just the symptoms.

Creating a Calm Environment: A calm and stable environment can significantly reduce the incidence of challenging behaviors. Excessive noise, clutter, or the presence of too many people can be overwhelming and disorienting for someone with Alzheimer's. Simplifying the environment, maintaining a routine, and providing a quiet space where the individual can retreat when feeling overwhelmed are all strategies that can create a sense of safety and reduce agitation.

Redirecting Attention: When a problematic behavior arises, one effective strategy is redirecting the individual's attention to a different activity or topic. This can be particularly useful when confrontation might escalate the behavior. For example, if the person becomes fixated on a particular subject, causing distress, gently guiding the conversation towards something more pleasant or engaging them in a different activity can help diffuse the situation. The key is to be subtle and gentle in the redirection, ensuring the individual feels respected and not manipulated.

Ensuring Safety: Safety is a paramount concern, especially for behaviors like wandering, which can put the individual at risk. Making the environment as safe as possible, using locks on doors and gates, and removing potential hazards can help prevent accidents. Additionally, using GPS devices or wearable alarms can provide an extra layer of security, giving caregivers peace of mind while respecting the individual's need for autonomy as much as possible.

Employing Compassionate Communication: Communication is crucial in all interactions, especially when managing difficult behaviors. Approaching the individual with empathy, attempting to understand their perspective, and speaking in a calm, reassuring tone can help prevent escalations. Acknowledging their feelings and providing reassurance that they are safe and cared for can often alleviate the anxiety or frustration driving the behavior.

Seeking Support: Finally, caregivers need to recognize when they need support. Managing challenging behaviors can be emotionally and physically draining, and no one should have to do it alone. Seeking advice from healthcare professionals, joining support groups, or arranging respite care can give caregivers the resources and breaks to recharge and continue providing care with patience and love.

Managing difficult behaviors in Alzheimer's requires empathy, patience, and creativity. By striving to understand the individual's needs, maintaining a supportive environment, and employing strategies tailored to the situation, caregivers can navigate these challenges with compassion and effectiveness, enhancing the quality of life for those they care for.

Coping with Caregiver Stress

Coping with caregiver stress is a critical aspect of the caregiving journey, especially for those caring for loved ones with Alzheimer's disease. The relentless nature of Alzheimer's, coupled with the gradual decline it brings, can place a significant emotional burden on caregivers. Managing this stress is important for the caregivers' well-being and the quality of care. Here are some strategies to help manage caregiver stress and maintain a healthy balance in life.

Seek Support: Finding a community of support is invaluable for caregivers. Joining a support group for Alzheimer's caregivers can offer a sense of belonging, understanding, and mutual support that is hard to find elsewhere. These groups provide a safe space to share experiences, challenges, and practical advice, reducing feelings of isolation and overwhelm. Whether it's through in-person meetings or online forums, connecting with others in similar situations can provide emotional relief and practical insights.

Take Time for Yourself: Caregiving can consume much time and energy, making it easy to neglect personal needs and interests. However, maintaining hobbies, social connections, and self-care practices is crucial for mental and emotional well-being. Activities that rejuvenate your spirit—reading, walking, meditation, or spending time with friends—can help recharge your emotional batteries. Remember, taking care of yourself is not a luxury; it's necessary to continue providing care.

Educate Yourself: Knowledge is a powerful tool in managing caregiver stress. Understanding Alzheimer's disease, its progression, and the challenges it brings can help set realistic expectations for both the caregiver and the person receiving care. Educating yourself about the disease can also empower you to make informed decisions about care strategies, anticipate and manage challenging behaviors, and communicate effectively with healthcare providers. Numerous resources, including books, online courses, and workshops, can enhance your knowledge and preparedness.

Consider Respite Care: Utilizing respite care services can offer caregivers a much-needed break and reduce the risk of burnout. Respite care can come in various forms, from in-home care services to adult daycare programs or short-term residential care. These services allow caregivers to take time for personal errands, rest, or leisure, secure knowing their loved one is in good hands. Regular breaks can help maintain a healthy perspective and resilience, making it easier to cope with the demands of caregiving.

Fostering Emotional Connections: Amid the practicalities of caregiving, it's important to nurture your loved one's emotional connection. Engaging in activities that bring joy and comfort, reminiscing about happy memories, or simply spending quiet time together can strengthen the bond between caregiver and recipient. These moments of connection can provide deep emotional sustenance for both parties, reminding them of the love and shared history that persists beyond the disease.

Recognizing the Emotional Journey: Caregiving for someone with Alzheimer's is as much an emotional journey as a physical and practical one. Acknowledging the emotional impact of caregiving and employing strategies to manage stress can lead to more fulfilling care experiences. Caregivers can find a sense of balance and resilience by seeking support, taking time for self-care, educating oneself, and utilizing respite care. Remember, you are not alone on this journey, and taking steps to care for your emotional well-being is essential for providing compassionate, effective care to your loved one.

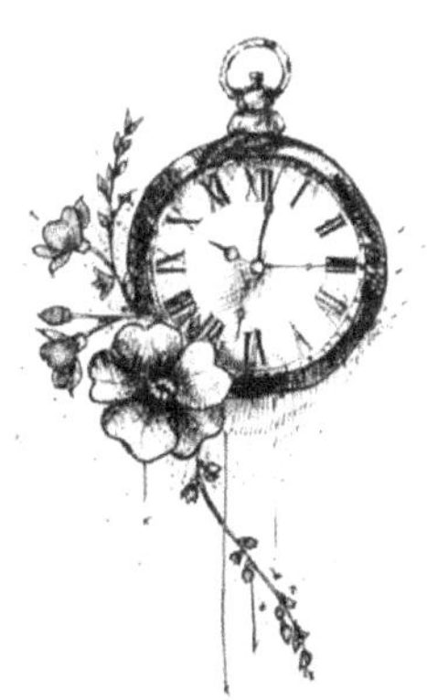

Chapter 3: Navigating the Early Stages of Alzheimer's Disease

The early stages of Alzheimer's disease represent a pivotal period that signifies the onset of a progressive journey, affecting not only those diagnosed with the condition but also profoundly impacting their families, loved ones, and caregivers. Navigating this initial phase with an informed perspective is essential for adapting to the changes ahead, ensuring the patient and their support network are prepared for the required challenges and adjustments.

What to Expect in the Early Stages of Alzheimer's Disease

In the early stages of Alzheimer's, individuals typically encounter subtle yet noticeable changes in cognitive functions. Symptoms may include:

Mild Memory Loss: This may manifest as forgetting recent conversations or events, misplacing items, or struggling to recall the names of new acquaintances. While these lapses can often be mistaken for normal aging, they are more frequent and disruptive in Alzheimer's.

Difficulty Finding Words: Language challenges become apparent, particularly in naming objects or expressing thoughts coherently. This can lead to pauses in conversation as the individual searches for the right words.

Challenges in Planning or Solving Problems: There may be noticeable difficulties in developing and following plans or working with numbers. Tasks that require organizational skills or managing finances may become overwhelming.

Changes in Mood and Behavior: Early stages can also bring changes in mood, including apathy, depression, or irritability. The person may show less interest in social activities or hobbies they once enjoyed.

Coping with Changes

As these symptoms gradually begin to impact daily life, both individuals with Alzheimer's and their caregivers need to develop strategies for managing these changes.

Understanding and adjusting to the early stages of Alzheimer's disease is a complex process that requires patience, compassion, and flexibility. By recognizing the signs, employing effective coping strategies, and accessing available resources, caregivers can provide meaningful support that respects the dignity and independence of their loved ones.

Providing Support in the Early Stages of Alzheimer's Disease

The early stages of Alzheimer's disease bring about changes that require adjustments in the way support is provided. Ensuring safety, maintaining independence, and planning for the future become paramount in creating a nurturing environment for your loved one.

Helping Your Loved One Maintain Independence: Preparation during the early stages of Alzheimer's disease can significantly impact the management and progression of the condition. Educating yourself and your family about Alzheimer's is a vital first step. Understanding the disease better will help you recognize symptoms early on and know what to expect as it progresses. This knowledge is essential for people with Alzheimer's and their loved ones, as it equips them to handle challenges more effectively.

Another critical aspect of preparation involves legal and financial planning. Discussing and making decisions regarding legal, financial, and healthcare matters early in the disease's progression is crucial. These discussions can help ensure that the wishes of the person with Alzheimer's are honored and that their affairs are in order, reducing stress and confusion for everyone involved later.

Creating a supportive environment is also key to managing Alzheimer's disease. Adjusting the living environment to make it safer and more comfortable can help manage symptoms and reduce risks associated with the disease. This might involve making physical modifications to the home or adapting daily routines to accommodate the changing needs of the person with Alzheimer's.

Finally, establishing a care team is essential. Building a network of family, friends, and medical professionals who can provide support will ease the burden of care as the disease progresses. This team approach to care can provide a comprehensive support system that addresses the physical, emotional, and social needs of the person with Alzheimer's and their caregivers.

Maintaining independence for as long as possible is vital for the self-esteem and overall well-being of someone living with Alzheimer's. Encouraging activity is one way to support your loved one. Supporting them in continuing their hobbies and interests by modifying activities to match their current abilities can provide a sense of normalcy and joy. Adaptive tools and technologies can also play a significant role in maintaining independence. Introducing tools such as medication reminders, simplified smartphones, or GPS trackers can help compensate for memory lapses and assist in daily living.

Empowering decision-making is another crucial strategy. Involving your loved one in decisions about their care and daily activities allows them to express their preferences and make choices whenever feasible. This involvement can help maintain their autonomy and dignity, positively contributing to their mental and emotional health.

Creating a Safe Environment at Home: As cognitive functions begin to decline in individuals with Alzheimer's, ensuring a safe home environment becomes increasingly crucial. This stage requires thoughtful modifications to the living space to minimize risks and enhance safety.

One of the first steps is removing hazards that could lead to falls or injuries. Simplifying the living space involves removing tripping hazards such as loose rugs, clutter, and unnecessary furniture. Installing grab bars in the bathroom can provide additional support and stability while ensuring the home is well-lit, which can help prevent accidents caused by poor visibility. These adjustments are essential for creating a safer living environment that accommodates the changing needs of someone with Alzheimer's.

Another important consideration is adapting the home to make it more navigable and understandable for your loved one. Using labels, signs, or color coding can help them navigate the home more easily and remember where things are stored. This can include labeling cabinets and drawers with words or pictures that indicate their contents or using different-colored tapes to mark the edges of steps to improve visibility. These adaptations can make a significant difference in the daily life of someone with Alzheimer's, helping them retain as much independence as possible.

Monitoring safety is also essential. Home safety technologies, such as automatic shut-off devices for appliances, can prevent accidents by automatically turning off devices that have been left on. Security systems that alert caregivers if their loved one wanders can also be invaluable, providing peace of mind and ensuring the safety of the individual with Alzheimer's. These technologies can be instrumental in managing the risks associated with cognitive decline, allowing for a safer and more secure home environment.

Planning for the Future: Early-stage Alzheimer's presents a critical window for planning and laying the groundwork for future care needs. This period is essential for making arrangements to ensure the well-being and support of the individual with Alzheimer's as the disease progresses.

Legal and financial planning is one of the first steps that should be taken during the early stages of Alzheimer's. Consulting with legal and financial advisors to set up necessary documents is crucial. This includes preparing wills, trusts, advanced healthcare directives, and a durable power of attorney. These documents will ensure that the person's wishes are respected and their affairs are managed according to their preferences. Taking these steps early can prevent a lot of stress and confusion in the future, making it easier for caregivers and family members to make decisions on behalf of their loved ones.

Care planning is another important aspect of preparing for the future. Beginning discussions about future care preferences early on allows individuals with Alzheimer's and their families to consider various options, such as home care, assisted living, or other long-term care solutions. Researching available services and support networks in the community can also provide valuable information and resources that will be beneficial. By having these conversations early, families can ensure that care decisions align with the individual's wishes and needs.

Establishing a relationship with healthcare providers specializing in Alzheimer's care is also vital. Planning regular check-ups and discussing the progression of the disease with medical professionals can help manage Alzheimer's more effectively. Healthcare providers can offer advice on medical interventions that may be beneficial and help families understand what to expect as the disease progresses.

Providing support in the early stages of Alzheimer's disease requires balancing safety and independence while also preparing for the future. By taking proactive steps early on, caregivers can better manage the progression of Alzheimer's, ensuring that their loved one receives the appropriate care and support they need as the disease advances. This preparation not only helps in adapting to the changing needs of someone with Alzheimer's but also provides peace of mind to families, knowing that plans are in place for the future.

Coping with Changes in Your Relationship with Your Loved One

The progression of Alzheimer's disease inevitably brings about changes in relationships, impacting the dynamics between those diagnosed and their caregivers. Understanding, adapting to these changes, and managing the associated emotions are key to providing compassionate care.

How Your Relationship Will Change: As Alzheimer's disease progresses, your loved one's cognitive decline and behavioral changes can significantly alter your relationship. Roles may reverse, with caregivers taking on responsibilities once managed by the person with Alzheimer's. Communication challenges can arise, making interactions more difficult. The person you once knew may seem different, affecting emotional connections and shared experiences.

Strategies for Maintaining a Positive Relationship: Maintaining a positive relationship with someone experiencing Alzheimer's requires adaptability, patience, and a strong focus on preserving the emotional connection despite the disease's changes. As the disease progresses, verbal communication may become more complex, making finding alternative ways to connect and express affection essential.

Focusing on nonverbal communication becomes increasingly important as verbal abilities decline. Simple gestures such as holding hands, a gentle touch, or a warm hug can convey love and reassurance. Music can also be a powerful tool for connection; sharing favorite songs or melodies can evoke memories and emotions, making it a meaningful activity to enjoy together. Engaging in shared activities, even simple ones, can maintain a sense of closeness and shared experience.

Adapting favorite activities to match the current abilities of a person with Alzheimer's is another way to maintain your bond. This might involve simplifying tasks or finding new ways to enjoy hobbies that were once loved. The goal is to find joy and satisfaction in doing things together, allowing you to create new memories even as the disease progresses.

Living in their reality is a compassionate approach significantly reducing frustrations and misunderstandings. Instead of correcting misconceptions or arguing with inaccurate statements, entering their reality by agreeing or playing along can lead to more positive interactions and decrease stress for the person with Alzheimer's and their caregiver.

Celebrating small moments and finding joy in the everyday can profoundly impact a relationship. These moments are precious, whether sharing a laugh, enjoying the outdoors, or listening to a favorite song. They help remind us that despite the challenges of Alzheimer's, the capacity for love, connection, and joy remains.

By embracing these strategies, caregivers can foster a nurturing and positive environment that honors the personhood of their loved one with Alzheimer's, ensuring that the journey ahead is filled with moments of connection and mutual respect.

Coping with Feelings of Grief and Loss: Grieving the gradual loss of the person you once knew, a phenomenon often referred to as "ambiguous loss," is a common and profoundly challenging experience for caregivers of individuals with Alzheimer's. This type of grief is unique because the loved one is physically present but psychologically changing or absent, leading to complex emotions and grief that can be difficult to process and articulate.

Acknowledging your feelings is a crucial first step in coping with ambiguous loss. Recognizing that it's normal to grieve the changes in your loved one and the impact these changes have on your relationship is important. This grief might manifest as sadness, anger, frustration, or many emotions. Accepting these feelings without judgment allows you to begin adapting to the new reality of your relationship.

Seeking support plays a vital role in navigating the emotional landscape of Alzheimer's caregiving. Connecting with friends, family, or others who are going through similar experiences can provide much-needed emotional relief and practical advice. Support groups, in-person or online, offer a space to share experiences and coping strategies. Counseling or therapy with a professional who understands the complexities of ambiguous loss can also be incredibly beneficial in helping you process these emotions.

Taking care of yourself is essential for your well-being and ensuring you can continue providing the best care for your loved one. Self-care activities include exercise, meditation, pursuing hobbies, or simply taking time for yourself. Maintaining your health through regular check-ups, eating well, and getting enough sleep is also critical. Self-care is not selfish; it's necessary to be a resilient caregiver.

Creating new ways to connect with your loved one can help maintain a sense of closeness despite the changes Alzheimer's brings. This might involve reminiscing through photos or stories, enjoying simple sensory activities like music, walking in nature, or finding new hobbies accessible to your loved one's current abilities. These activities can offer comfort and joy to both of you, fostering a positive relationship amidst the challenges.

Coping with the changes in your relationship as your loved one progresses through the stages of Alzheimer's requires compassion, resilience, and adaptability. By focusing on maintaining a positive relationship, adapting to new ways of connecting, and taking care of your emotional and physical well-being, you can navigate these changes with grace and strength, ensuring that you and your loved one experience moments of connection and joy amidst the challenges.

Make a Difference with Your Review

Unlock the Power of Generosity

"Helping one person might not change the whole world, but it could change the world for one person." - Anonymous.

Helping others without expecting anything in return can make us feel happier and more fulfilled. So, if we can help someone during our time together, you bet we'll take it!

Here's something I'd like to ask you...

Would you help someone you've never met, even if you knew you wouldn't get anything in return?

Imagine someone who's just like you or who you were before. They're looking for ways to understand and help someone they care about, maybe someone facing Alzheimer's, but they're unsure where to start.

Our mission is to make *The 5 Stages of Alzheimer's* a helpful resource for everyone. Everything we do is about that mission. But we can't do it alone—we need to reach... well, everyone.

And that's where you come in. You see, most people decide which book to read based on what others say. So, on behalf of someone out there who needs guidance, I'm asking:

Please leave a review for this book.

It won't cost you a dime and will take less than a minute, but your review could be a game-changer. It might help:

...another family navigates the challenges of Alzheimer's with hope. ...a caregiver finds new ways to support and connect. ...an individual understands their loved one better. ...a community come together to support each other. ...a heart finds peace in tough times.

To spread a little happiness and make a difference, take a moment to:

Leave your review.

Just scan the QR code below to share your thoughts:

https://www.amazon.com/review/create-
review/?ie=UTF8&channel=glance-detail&asin=B0CYQPKNWV

If the thought of helping someone out there warms your heart, you're our kind of person. Welcome to the club. You're one of us now.

I can't wait to help you learn more about Alzheimer's care with even more understanding and compassion. The advice and insights in the following chapters will be worth it.

Thank you from the bottom of my heart. Now, let's get back to learning and helping together.

Your biggest fan,

G.M. Grace

PS - Remember: Sharing valuable information makes you a valuable person to someone else. If you believe this book can help another reader, caregiver, or family member, pass it along. They'll appreciate it, and so will you.

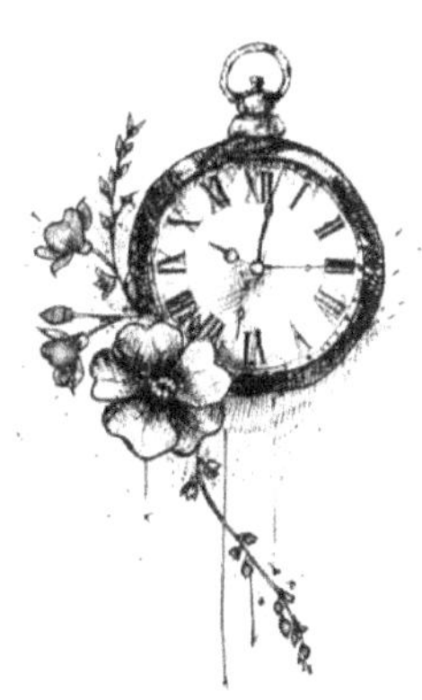

Chapter 4: Navigating the Middle Stages of Alzheimer's Disease

Understanding the Middle Stages

The middle stages of Alzheimer's disease mark a significant transition in the progression of the condition. This period can be particularly challenging for the individual experiencing the disease and their caregivers. Understanding what to expect, preparing for the challenges, and developing strategies to cope with changes are essential steps in navigating this phase.

What to Expect in the Middle Stages

In the middle stages of Alzheimer's, symptoms become more pronounced. Memory loss worsens, and changes in cognition and physical abilities become more evident. Individuals may have difficulty performing daily tasks, exhibit changes in personality and behavior, experience confusion about events or their environment, and struggle with language and communication. It's common for individuals to exhibit repetitive behaviors, restlessness, and sometimes agitation or aggression.

How to Prepare for the Middle Stages

Preparation for the middle stages involves both practical and emotional readiness.

Modify the Living Environment: Adjust the home to improve safety and accessibility. This may include adding locks, safety rails, and removing hazards.

Establish a Routine: Consistent daily routines can help reduce confusion and provide stability.

Plan for Increased Care Needs: Assess the evolving care needs and consider options for additional support, such as in-home care services or adult day care programs.

Educate Yourself: Learn more about Alzheimer's-related behaviors and communication strategies to better interact with and support your loved one.

Coping with Changes in Memory and Behavior

Coping with the advancing symptoms requires patience, understanding, and flexibility.

Communication Strategies: Use simple, clear sentences and visual cues to aid understanding. Always approach with calmness and patience.

Behavioral Management: Identify triggers for difficult behaviors. Create a calm environment and find activities to soothe and engage your loved one.

Support for Memory Loss: Use memory aids and establish routines to help your loved one navigate their day with less confusion.

Seek Support: Connect with caregiver support groups and resources for emotional support and practical advice. Taking care of your mental and emotional health is crucial during this demanding stage.

Navigating the middle stages of Alzheimer's disease requires a comprehensive approach that addresses the increasing care needs, behavioral changes, and emotional challenges faced by individuals and their caregivers. By understanding what to expect, preparing adequately, and employing effective coping strategies, it is possible to manage the symptoms and maintain quality of life during this phase of the disease.

Providing Support in the Middle Stages

As Alzheimer's disease progresses into the middle stages, the need for comprehensive care and support becomes more critical. Here, we delve into ways to help maintain the independence of your loved one, ensure their environment is safe, and plan for the future as the disease progresses.

Helping Your Loved One Maintain Independence

Maintaining a sense of independence for as long as possible is crucial for the dignity and self-esteem of someone living with Alzheimer's.

Encourage Participation in Daily Tasks: To foster a sense of accomplishment, allow your loved one to engage in simple daily activities or hobbies they enjoy and can safely perform, such as setting the table or gardening.

Provide Choices: Offer limited choices to help them maintain control, such as choosing between two outfits or choosing meals.

Creating a Safe Environment at Home

As cognitive abilities decline, ensuring the home is safe becomes paramount.

Conduct a Safety Check: Regularly review the home for hazards—loose rugs, poor lighting, or obstacles that could cause trips and falls—and make necessary adjustments.

Implement Safety Measures: Install locks on cabinets containing harmful substances, use automatic shut-off devices for kitchen appliances, and consider a monitoring system to alert you if your loved one is wandering.

Organize the Living Space: To minimize confusion and anxiety, keep the environment clutter-free and organized. Labeling cabinets and doors can help your loved one navigate their space more efficiently.

Planning for the Future

Navigating the middle stages of Alzheimer's disease is a pivotal period for caregivers and their loved ones. During this time, the disease's progression becomes more evident, presenting new challenges and necessitating thoughtful planning for the future. Here's a closer look at essential steps to consider during this critical phase:

Long-Term Care Options: The middle stages of Alzheimer's are an opportune time to explore long-term care options. This might involve looking into assisted living facilities and memory care units or considering in-home care services. It's beneficial to involve your loved one in these discussions to the extent possible, respecting their preferences and autonomy. Researching and visiting potential facilities or interviewing in-home care providers early can help make a more informed decision when the time for transition arrives.

Build a Support Network: Establishing and maintaining a solid support network is crucial for caregivers and their loved ones. This network can include family, friends, Alzheimer's support groups, and professional caregivers. A robust support system offers emotional solace and practical assistance, easing the burden of caregiving. Respite care, whether through professional services or informal arrangements with family and friends, allows caregivers to take necessary breaks and helps prevent burnout.

Providing support during the middle stages of Alzheimer's involves a careful balance between ensuring safety and promoting as much independence as possible. By addressing any legal and financial affairs not already taken care of, considering future care needs, and building a supportive network, caregivers can better manage the challenges of this phase. It's essential to adapt to the evolving needs of your loved one, ensuring that the care environment is secure, supportive, and respectful of their dignity. Planning and preparation during these middle stages lay the foundation for navigating Alzheimer's with compassion and resilience, ensuring the best possible quality of life for your loved one.

Strategies for Maintaining a Positive Relationship with Your Loved One

Maintaining a positive relationship with a loved one who has Alzheimer's disease presents unique challenges, requiring a deep well of patience, empathy, and adaptability from caregivers. Here are some strategies to foster a nurturing and positive connection throughout the progression of the disease:

Focus on the Present: With Alzheimer's, the ability to recall recent interactions gradually fades. However, the emotional impact of positive experiences can linger. Cherish the moments of joy, laughter, and connection you share with your loved one now, recognizing the value of the present. Even if the details of these moments might not be remembered, the feelings of love and happiness can still comfort your loved one.

Adapt Communication: As Alzheimer's progresses, effective communication with your loved one requires adjustments. Simplify your language, speak clearly, and use shorter sentences to make it easier for them to understand. Non-verbal cues, such as eye contact, smiles, and gentle touches, can also convey messages of love and reassurance. Remaining patient and positive in your interactions helps create a supportive atmosphere that can reduce frustration and confusion for your loved one.

Engage in Enjoyable Activities: Identifying activities you can enjoy together and adapting them to your loved one's current abilities can enhance quality time together. Music has a universal appeal and can often reach individuals with Alzheimer's in profound ways, evoking memories and emotions. Art activities like painting or coloring provide a creative outlet and a sense of accomplishment. Nature walks or simply spending time outdoors can be calming and provide sensory stimulation. Tailoring these activities to your loved one's interests and capabilities can lead to enjoyable and fulfilling experiences for both of you.

Practice Empathy. Putting yourself in your loved one's shoes can provide invaluable insights into their world experience. Alzheimer's can make the world confusing and sometimes frightening. You reinforce your emotional bond by acknowledging and validating their feelings, even if their perceptions differ from reality. Empathy allows you to respond to their needs and emotions in a way that affirms their dignity and worth.

Maintaining a positive relationship amidst the challenges of Alzheimer's is an ongoing process that evolves with the disease. By focusing on the present, adapting communication strategies, engaging in enjoyable activities, and practicing empathy, caregivers can navigate the complexities of Alzheimer's with compassion and resilience. This approach not only supports the well-being of the individual with Alzheimer's but also enriches the caregiving experience, fostering moments of connection that become precious memories.

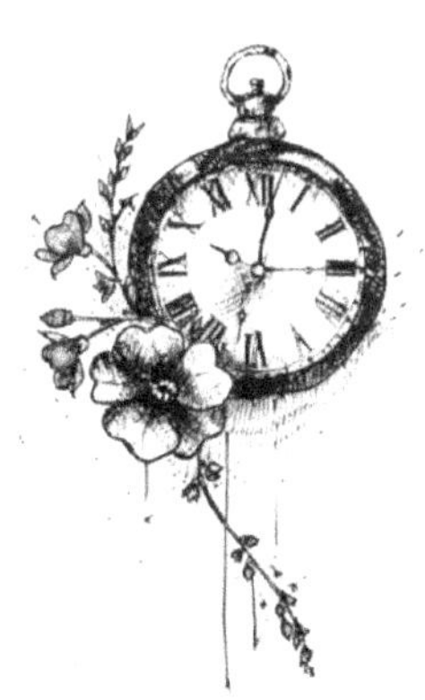

Chapter Five: Navigating Late-Stage Alzheimer's Disease

Understanding Late-Stage

The late stage of Alzheimer's disease represents the most advanced phase of this condition. It's a time that requires significant adjustments and preparations, both emotionally and practically, for caregivers and families. Understanding what to expect, how to prepare, and ways to cope with changes are essential for providing compassionate care during this challenging time.

What to Expect in Late-Stage

In late-stage Alzheimer's, individuals may lose the ability to communicate verbally and require full-time assistance with daily activities. Physical abilities decline, leading to the need for help with walking, sitting, and eventually, swallowing. Cognitive skills continue to deteriorate, losing awareness of one's environment and experiences. It's

93

also common for health complications to arise, such as infections, due to decreased mobility and swallowing difficulties.

How to Prepare for Late-Stage

Preparing for the late stages of Alzheimer's disease is a multifaceted process that encompasses medical and emotional considerations. Each aspect is crucial for ensuring that the individual receives the care and support needed during this challenging time while also addressing family members' and caregivers' needs and well-being. Here's a closer look at these critical considerations:

Medical Care Planning: In the late stages of Alzheimer's, medical care often focuses on comfort and quality of life rather than curative treatments. Establishing a care team specialized in end-of-life care is essential. This team might include doctors, nurses, hospice care professionals, and other specialists experienced in managing the symptoms associated with advanced Alzheimer's. They work together to provide pain management, symptom relief, and emotional support, ensuring the individual's comfort and dignity.

Emotional Support: The emotional and psychological impact of caring for someone in the late stages of Alzheimer's can be profound. Seeking support for both caregivers and family members is vital. This support can come from counseling, Alzheimer's support groups, or spiritual advisors, providing a space to express feelings, share experiences, and receive guidance on coping with grief and loss. Such support networks offer comfort and reassurance during this challenging journey.

Home Safety and Comfort: Adapting the living environment to meet the evolving needs of someone with late-stage Alzheimer's is essential for their safety and comfort. This might involve modifications to the home to prevent falls, ensuring easy access to the bed and bathroom, and using specialized equipment like hospital beds, wheelchairs, and adaptive utensils. The goal is to create a safe, comfortable, accessible living space that accommodates individual needs and promotes well-being.

Preparing for the late stages of Alzheimer's disease requires thoughtful consideration and planning across these critical areas. Families and caregivers can provide the most compassionate and comprehensive care possible by addressing medical care, emotional support, and home safety and comfort. This preparation benefits the individual with Alzheimer's and provides peace of mind and support for those who care for them, ensuring they are not alone in navigating the challenges ahead.

Coping with Changes in Memory and Behavior

Coping with the late stages of Alzheimer's disease presents unique challenges, as individuals experience significant declines in memory and behavior, alongside an increased dependency on caregivers for daily activities. This phase demands a gentle, patient approach focused on comfort, quality of life, and maintaining an emotional connection despite profound changes. Here are strategies to navigate this delicate stage:

Nonverbal Communication: As verbal communication diminishes, nonverbal cues become crucial in understanding the needs of a loved one with late-stage Alzheimer's. Observing facial expressions, body language, and other indicators of discomfort or pain is essential for providing appropriate care. Attention to these signals can help address the person's needs effectively, even when they can't articulate them.

Maintain Emotional Connection: Maintaining an emotional connection becomes paramount during this stage. Simple acts of kindness, such as holding hands, playing their favorite music, reading aloud, or sitting beside them, can provide immense comfort and reassurance. These actions remind your loved one of your presence and love, offering solace even as cognitive abilities decline.

Manage Physical Needs: Collaborating with healthcare professionals is key to managing the physical challenges that arise during late-stage Alzheimer's. This includes addressing pain management, ensuring comfort, and finding creative solutions for nutritional needs, especially as difficulties with eating and swallowing emerge. Tailoring care strategies to the individual's changing needs is vital for their well-being.

Self-Care for Caregivers: The intensity of caregiving during the late stages of Alzheimer's can significantly toll caregivers, both emotionally and physically. Caregivers must prioritize their well-being. This can involve seeking respite care to take necessary breaks, relying on a support network of family, friends, or support groups, and engaging in self-care practices to maintain their health. Recognizing the need for help and allowing oneself to receive it is essential for sustaining the capacity to provide care.

Navigating the late stages of Alzheimer's disease is undoubtedly challenging, requiring a balance of compassion, patience, and practicality. Families can navigate this journey gracefully by focusing on non-verbal communication, maintaining emotional connections, managing physical needs, and emphasizing caregiver self-care. Understanding what to expect and preparing for the changes can help ensure that the final stages of Alzheimer's are marked by dignity, comfort, and a deep sense of care.

Providing support in Late-Stage

Providing care during the late stages of Alzheimer's disease is a profound responsibility that requires a deep commitment to ensuring the patient's comfort, dignity, and quality of life. As caregivers navigate this challenging phase, several strategies can be employed to offer the best possible support:

Helping Your Loved One Maintain Independence

In the late stages of Alzheimer's, maintaining independence focuses on preserving the individual's dignity and enhancing their quality of life.

Support Residual Abilities: Recognizing and encouraging any remaining abilities is vital. This could involve activities that elicit responses, such as playing favorite pieces of music, providing objects with varied tactile sensations, or sharing photographs that may prompt a smile or a moment of recognition. Celebrating these small victories can significantly impact the individual's sense of self and well-being.

Personalized Care: Tailoring care to the individual's long-standing preferences respects their dignity and personal history. This could mean playing their favorite music, adhering to established routines for daily activities, or incorporating their favorite foods safely and flexibly. Personalized care helps maintain a connection to their identity and past preferences.

Creating a Safe Environment at Home

As Alzheimer's progresses, ensuring a safe living environment becomes increasingly important due to decreased mobility and awareness.

Adapt the Home Environment: Modifying the home can significantly reduce the risk of falls and injuries. This might include installing bed rails, using pressure mattresses to prevent bedsores, and arranging furniture to accommodate mobility aids. Creating a navigable and secure environment prevents accidents and promotes comfort.

Monitor Health Closely: Vigilance in observing signs of pain, discomfort, or potential health issues is crucial. This includes monitoring for signs of infections or other medical conditions that may require prompt attention. Working closely with healthcare providers ensures that concerns are addressed swiftly and effectively.

Planning for the Future by Making the Decision to Place or Not to Place Your Loved One in an Outside Facility

One of the most challenging decisions in late-stage Alzheimer's care involves considering whether to move the individual into a specialized care facility.

Evaluate Care Needs: Assessing the ability to meet the increasing care needs at home is crucial. This includes considering caregiving's physical, emotional, and logistical aspects and whether these can be sustainably managed in the home setting.

Consider Quality of Life: Reflecting on the quality of life provided at home versus in a specialized care facility is essential. Facilities may offer professional care, social engagement opportunities, and resources that might be challenging to replicate at home.

Seek Professional Advice: Consulting healthcare professionals, social workers, and organizations specializing in Alzheimer's care can provide valuable insights into the available options and help guide the decision-making process.

Discuss with Family: Engaging in open discussions with family members about care preferences, concerns, and the practicalities of different care options is important. The goal should be a decision considering the best interests and well-being of the individual with Alzheimer's.

Deciding on care placement is a profoundly personal and complex process, influenced by various factors, including the caregiver's capacity, financial resources, and the availability of quality care facilities. Regardless of the decision, it should be approached with empathy and a focus on what is best for the individual's dignity and quality of life in the late stages of Alzheimer's.

Coping with Changes in Your Relationship with Your Loved One

Navigating the journey of Alzheimer's disease profoundly impacts the relationships between patients and their caregivers, particularly as the disease progresses into its late stages. This progression can significantly transform the dynamics of these relationships, affecting both emotional connections and day-to-day interactions.

How Your Relationship Will Change

As Alzheimer's disease advances, the cognitive and physical abilities of the person with Alzheimer's decline, leading to a fundamental shift in the relationship. Caregivers often take on roles and responsibilities once managed by their loved ones, which can alter the relationship dynamic. Communication challenges become more pronounced, making it difficult to connect in the ways you once did. This can create a profound sense of loss and mourning for the relationship as it was before the disease, as the person you know seems increasingly distant.

Strategies for Maintaining a Positive Relationship with Your Loved One

Despite these challenges, there are strategies to maintain a positive relationship with your loved one during Alzheimer's:

Focus on Non-Verbal Communication: As verbal communication skills diminish, other forms of connection, such as physical touch, shared activities, and simply being present, become invaluable in conveying love and support.

Adapt to Their Reality: Trying to correct or confront the altered perceptions of a person with Alzheimer's can lead to frustration for both of you. Instead, entering their reality and engaging with them within it can foster more peaceful and meaningful interactions.

Celebrate the Good Moments: It's important to cherish the moments of clarity and joy, no matter how brief. These moments can offer significant comfort and connection.

Create a Legacy: Honoring the life and memories of your loved one through actions like compiling a photo album or creating a memory box can help celebrate their identity beyond the disease.

Coping with the evolving relationship with a loved one with late-stage Alzheimer's is a profoundly personal journey. By adapting, maintaining connection, and managing grief with compassion, caregivers can navigate these changes, ensuring that the bond with their loved one remains a source of strength and love.

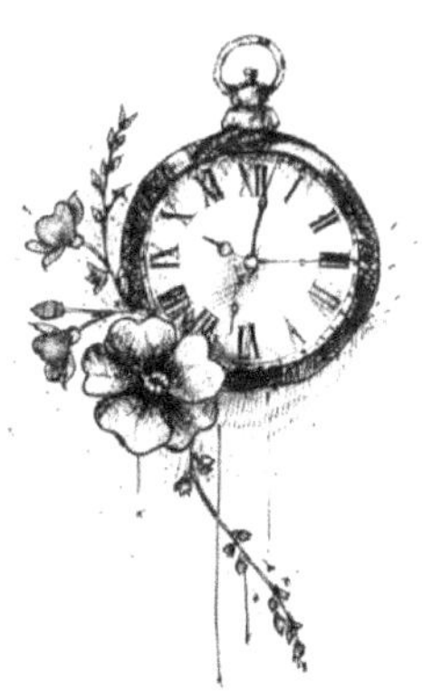

Chapter Six – Legal and Financial Planning

Understanding Legal and Financial Planning

What is Legal and Financial Planning?

Legal and financial planning involves carefully considering and arranging legal matters and financial affairs to ensure the well-being and protection of individuals, particularly in the context of Alzheimer's disease. This planning encompasses a variety of legal documents, such as wills, trusts, powers of attorney, and advance directives, as well as financial strategies to manage assets, healthcare expenses, and long-term care costs.

Why are Legal and Financial Planning Important?

Legal and financial planning are indispensable for individuals and families navigating the complexities of Alzheimer's disease. This planning is critical for several reasons, each pivotal in ensuring the well-being and security of the affected individual and their loved ones.

Decision-making: As Alzheimer's disease progresses, cognitive decline can significantly impair an individual's ability to make informed decisions about their finances, healthcare, and personal affairs. Early establishment of legal documents like a durable power of attorney and a healthcare proxy ensures that trusted individuals are appointed to make decisions on behalf of the affected person. This is crucial for maintaining continuity in financial management and healthcare choices that align with the individual's wishes.

Asset protection: The financial vulnerability of individuals with Alzheimer's disease cannot be overstated. They are at increased risk of exploitation, fraud, and mismanagement of their assets. Proper legal and financial planning, including using trusts and careful beneficiary designations, offers a safeguard against such risks. These strategies ensure that assets are protected and utilized according to the individual's intentions, particularly regarding funding long-term care and supporting their quality of life.

Healthcare management: The trajectory of Alzheimer's disease often requires comprehensive medical care and support services, ranging from daily living assistance to specialized healthcare. Planning facilitates access to quality care and ensures the individual's treatment preferences are respected. This is achieved through legal documents such as advance directives and living wills, which articulate the individual's wishes regarding medical treatments and end-of-life care. These documents help avoid unnecessary interventions and focus on comfort and dignity.

Family harmony: Alzheimer's disease can place immense stress on families, not just emotionally but also in terms of managing care and financial responsibilities. Without clear guidance, disputes can arise over care decisions, financial management, and inheritance issues. By establishing clear legal and financial plans, families can mitigate these tensions. Such plans set forth explicit instructions for care preferences, asset distribution, and the roles and responsibilities of each family member, fostering understanding and cooperation among loved ones.

In essence, legal and financial planning for Alzheimer's disease is not just about managing assets and healthcare decisions; it's about ensuring the affected individual's dignity, preferences, and security while minimizing the emotional and financial strain on their families. It paves the way for a structured approach to care, preserves family relationships, and protects the legacy and wishes of those facing the challenges of Alzheimer's.

How to Get Started with Legal and Financial Planning

Engaging in legal and financial planning is an essential step for individuals diagnosed with Alzheimer's disease and their families. This proactive approach helps navigate the complexities associated with the disease, ensuring that immediate and future needs are addressed. Here's a guide on how to get started:

Consult with Professionals: The journey begins with experienced professionals specializing in elder law and financial planning for Alzheimer's care. Attorneys in this niche can provide crucial advice on legal strategies and help draft necessary documents, ensuring they are tailored to your loved one's unique situation. Similarly, financial advisors familiar with Alzheimer's planning can offer insights on managing and allocating financial resources effectively to cover long-term care needs. These experts can assess the situation holistically, offering personalized recommendations that align with your goals.

Identify Key Documents

A solid legal and financial plan includes several key documents:

A **Will** ensures that assets are distributed according to your loved one's wishes upon passing.

Trusts can provide a more controlled distribution of assets and help manage or avoid estate taxes.

Powers of Attorney allow your loved one to designate someone to make financial and healthcare decisions on their behalf if unable to do so.

Advance Directives communicate their wishes regarding end-of-life care.

Guardianship or Conservatorship Arrangements may be necessary if your loved one hasn't designated someone to make decisions for them and they cannot manage their affairs.

Understanding the purpose and importance of each document is crucial for effective planning.

Assess Financial Resources: Careful assessment of financial resources is vital. This includes current assets, income sources, insurance policies, and retirement savings. Knowing what the person with Alzheimer's has is the first step in planning how to use these resources to cover future care needs and other expenses. This assessment will form the basis of the financial planning, helping to ensure that resources are allocated to best support long-term care needs and preferences.

Plan for the Future: With a clear understanding of the legal options and financial resources, you can develop a comprehensive plan that addresses immediate and future concerns. This plan should consider long-term care preferences, potential housing options, and legacy planning. It's important to regularly review and update this plan to reflect any changes in the circumstances, health, financial situation, or goals.

By taking these steps, individuals and families dealing with Alzheimer's disease can create a robust framework to manage the legal and financial challenges posed by the disease. This planning ensures that the individual's care needs and preferences are met. It provides peace of mind and security for the future, allowing families to focus on quality care and making the most of their time together.

Legal Planning

Power of Attorney

A Power of Attorney (POA) is an essential legal instrument, especially for individuals diagnosed with Alzheimer's disease or those at risk of becoming incapacitated. It ensures that a trusted individual can manage their financial and legal affairs if they can no longer decide for themselves. Here are key aspects to consider:

Durable Power of Attorney: Unlike a standard POA, which becomes invalid if the principal becomes incapacitated, a durable power of attorney remains in effect during incapacitation. This durability is crucial for Alzheimer's patients, as it ensures continuous management of their affairs without the need for court intervention to establish guardianship or conservatorship.

Scope of Authority: The agent or attorney-in-fact appointed through a POA has broad authority to manage the principal's financial matters. This can include paying bills, managing bank accounts, making investment decisions, selling property, and handling tax matters. The powers granted can be tailored within the POA document to fit the principal's needs and preferences.

Choosing an Agent: Selecting an agent is one of the most critical decisions when establishing a POA. The agent should implicitly be someone the principal trusts, such as a close family member or longtime friend. It's important that the chosen agent is willing to take on the responsibility, can manage financial affairs competently, and will always act in the principal's best interests.

Instructions and Preferences: While the POA grants the agent authority to make decisions, it can also include specific instructions or preferences regarding how certain matters should be handled. This can guide the agent and help ensure that the principal's wishes are followed as closely as possible.

Early Preparation: Given the progressive nature of Alzheimer's disease, it's advisable to establish a durable power of attorney early in the diagnosis. This ensures that the individual can actively participate in selecting their agent and drafting the document, which accurately reflects their wishes.

A durable power of attorney provides peace of mind to individuals with Alzheimer's and their families, knowing that their financial and legal affairs will be handled according to their wishes, even if they cannot manage these matters themselves. This proactive step is crucial in comprehensive care and estate planning, allowing for smoother management of the individual's affairs and minimizing potential conflicts or legal complications.

Guardianship

Guardianship, or conservatorship as it is known in some jurisdictions, is an important legal mechanism designed to protect individuals who can no longer manage their affairs, such as those with advanced stages of Alzheimer's disease. This process is especially critical when planning documents like a power of attorney are not in place or when the person appointed under such documents can no longer perform their duties effectively. Here's a deeper look into the guardianship process and its implications:

When a guardianship is established, the court appoints a guardian to make decisions on behalf of the incapacitated person, referred to as the ward. This appointment is a significant responsibility, encompassing decisions related to the ward's finances, healthcare, and personal well-being. The guardian's decisions must align with the ward's best interests, ensuring their health, safety, and financial security.

Establishing guardianship involves petitioning the court, typically followed by a formal assessment or evaluation to confirm the individual's incapacity. This process can be emotionally challenging for families, as it involves legal proceedings and, often, discussions about the personal and medical condition of their loved one. Due to its complexity and the need for court oversight, guardianship can incur substantial legal fees. It requires the guardian to provide regular reports to the court about the ward's status and how decisions are being made.

Given these considerations, exploring all other options, such as establishing a durable power of attorney and healthcare directives, is generally advisable before pursuing guardianship. These planning tools allow individuals to designate someone they trust to manage their affairs should they become incapacitated, offering a more straightforward and less invasive way to ensure their needs are met. However, when such documents are not in place or are insufficient, guardianship becomes crucial for providing care and protection.

Guardianship is intended to safeguard the rights and well-being of individuals who cannot care for themselves. Still, it also involves significant responsibilities and legal complexities for the appointed guardian. For families navigating the challenges of Alzheimer's disease, understanding the guardianship process and its implications is essential for making informed decisions about the care and protection of their loved ones. It underscores the importance of early planning and open discussions about future care preferences and legal arrangements.

Advance Directives

Advance directives serve as a critical component of planning for individuals with Alzheimer's disease, ensuring that their healthcare preferences are respected and followed significantly as their ability to communicate diminishes. These legal documents allow individuals to maintain autonomy over their medical treatment and end-of-life care decisions. Here's a closer look at the common types of advance directives and their significance:

Living Will: A living will is a document that outlines the types of medical treatments and life-sustaining measures an individual wishes to accept or refuse if faced with a terminal illness or irreversible condition and cannot communicate their decisions. It might include directives regarding ventilators, artificial nutrition and hydration, resuscitation efforts, and the extent of palliative care to be administered. This document serves as a guide for healthcare providers and family members, helping to ensure that the individual's end-of-life care preferences are understood and honored.

Healthcare Proxy or Durable Power of Attorney for Healthcare: This document allows an individual to appoint a trusted person as their healthcare agent or proxy, granting them the authority to make healthcare decisions on the individual's behalf if they are incapacitated or otherwise unable to make decisions for themselves. The appointed agent is responsible for making medical decisions that align with the individual's preferences and values, covering various treatments and interventions. The designation of a healthcare proxy ensures that someone knows the individual's wishes and is legally empowered to advocate for those wishes in medical situations.

Establishing advance directives encourages individuals and their families to engage in meaningful conversations about healthcare preferences, values, and end-of-life wishes. These discussions are essential for ensuring the appointed healthcare proxy fully understands the individual's desires and is prepared to act in their best interest.

Incorporating advance directives into a comprehensive care strategy for Alzheimer's provides clarity and guidance for medical professionals and caregivers. It offers reassurance and peace of mind to the individual and their loved ones. Knowing that plans are in place for managing healthcare decisions according to the individual's wishes can alleviate some of the emotional burdens associated with navigating the complexities of Alzheimer's care.

It's important for individuals, especially those diagnosed with Alzheimer's or at risk of developing the disease, to complete advance directives while they still can make informed decisions. Legal advice and guidance from healthcare professionals can ensure that these documents are appropriately executed and reflect the individual's specific wishes regarding their care.

Financial Planning

Budgeting for Care

Budgeting for care in the context of Alzheimer's disease is an essential component of financial planning for affected individuals and their families. Given the progressive nature of Alzheimer's, the need for specialized care and support services escalates over time, leading to increased financial demands. Here are strategic steps to effectively budget for Alzheimer's care:

Assess Current and Anticipated Costs: Start by evaluating the current expenses related to the individual's care. This includes costs for medical care, medications, necessary home modifications for safety and accessibility, and caregiver support, whether professional or informal. It's important also to anticipate future costs, which can escalate significantly as the disease progresses. Consider potential needs for more intensive care options, such as assisted living facilities or skilled nursing care, and how these might impact financial planning.

Create a Comprehensive Budget: Develop a budget that comprehensively accounts for all sources of income and expenses. This should include fixed income sources such as pensions, Social Security benefits, and other investments or savings. Also, consider financial assistance programs for which the individual may be eligible. Allocate funds to cover essential expenses, prioritizing healthcare, housing, food, transportation, and personal care needs. This budget should be a roadmap for managing finances to ensure continuous access to necessary care services.

Consider Cost-Effective Care Options: To manage costs more effectively, explore various care options that might offer savings without compromising the quality of care. In some cases, family members' care, with support from community-based organizations, can be a cost-effective alternative to professional home care services. Additionally, some community organizations offer meal delivery, transportation, and day programs at reduced costs or on a sliding scale based on income.

Plan for Unexpected Expenses: One of the challenges of financial planning for Alzheimer's care is the potential for unexpected expenses, which can arise from emergency medical needs, sudden changes in care requirements, or unforeseen home repairs. To mitigate these risks, establish an emergency savings account specifically designated for such expenses or ensure the budget includes a buffer to absorb financial shocks without compromising the individual's care or family's financial stability.

Proactively budgeting for Alzheimer's care allows individuals and families to navigate the financial complexities of the disease with greater confidence. Families can create a sustainable financial plan by understanding the full scope of current and future care needs, leveraging all available income sources, and planning for the unexpected. This plan not only supports the ongoing care requirements of the individual with Alzheimer's but also helps maintain financial health and access to necessary resources throughout the disease.

Long-Term Care Insurance

Long-term care insurance is an essential consideration for individuals planning for the financial aspects of Alzheimer's disease and other long-term care needs. This type of insurance can help cover the costs of services that assist with activities of daily living (ADLs), skilled nursing care, and memory care services, which are crucial for individuals with Alzheimer's disease. Here's a detailed look at the key considerations when evaluating long-term care insurance:

Coverage Options: It's crucial to thoroughly evaluate different long-term care insurance policies to understand the breadth and depth of coverage they offer. This includes looking at the benefit amounts—how much the policy will pay per day or month for care services—and the range of covered services, such as in-home care, assisted living, nursing home care, and specialized memory care. Also, consider the policy's elimination period (the waiting period before benefits start) and whether the policy offers inflation protection to ensure the benefit amount keeps pace with the rising cost of care over time.

Premium Costs: The affordability of long-term care insurance premiums is a significant factor. Premiums are influenced by several factors, including the applicant's age at the time of purchase, health status, and the chosen coverage options. Generally, premiums are lower for younger, healthier individuals. It's also important to consider the impact of potential premium increases over time and how they fit into your financial planning. Assessing whether the premiums are manageable within your current and projected income and financial resources is essential.

Policy Features: Understanding the specific features and limitations of a long-term care insurance policy is critical. This includes knowing what triggers the policy benefits—typically a defined level of disability or the inability to perform a certain number of ADLs. Waiting periods or the amount of time before benefits can be accessed after qualifying for care and any exclusions for pre-existing conditions should also be reviewed to ensure the policy meets your needs and expectations.

Integration with Other Resources: Long-term care insurance should be considered part of a broader financial strategy for covering care costs. This involves understanding how it can complement other financial resources you may have, such as Medicaid (which may cover long-term care for those who meet eligibility criteria), veterans' benefits, or personal savings and investments. Integrating long-term care insurance with these resources can help create a more comprehensive and effective plan for financing long-term care needs.

Given the high costs associated with Alzheimer's care and the likelihood of requiring long-term care services, long-term care insurance can offer valuable financial protection. However, it's essential to carefully evaluate policy options, consider how a policy fits into your overall financial planning, and review the specific terms and conditions to ensure they align with your circumstances and care planning goals. Consulting with a financial planner or insurance specialist who understands long-term care insurance can provide valuable insights and help guide your decision-making process.

Medicaid

Navigating Medicaid for long-term care, especially for individuals with Alzheimer's disease, involves understanding complex eligibility criteria, planning strategies, and the range of services covered. This understanding is crucial for accessing the necessary care while preserving financial stability. Here's a closer look at critical considerations for Medicaid eligibility and planning:

Eligibility Criteria: Medicaid's eligibility for long-term care benefits is determined by specific income and asset limits that vary by state. Applicants must meet these financial criteria to qualify for benefits. Additionally, Medicaid employs a "look-back period," typically five years, during which all financial transactions are scrutinized. This prevents individuals from transferring assets solely to meet Medicaid's eligibility requirements. Understanding these rules is essential to plan effectively for Medicaid eligibility without inadvertently disqualifying oneself.

Medicaid Planning Strategies: Working with a qualified elder law attorney can be invaluable in navigating these financial eligibility criteria. These professionals can help develop strategies to protect assets while ensuring legal eligibility for Medicaid. Common strategies include using certain types of trusts, asset transfers (subject to the look-back period rules), purchasing annuities designed to comply with Medicaid rules, and utilizing protections for the spouse of a nursing home resident, such as the Community Spouse Resource Allowance. These strategies must be employed carefully to avoid penalties and ensure they align with Medicaid regulations.

Medicaid Application Process: Applying for Medicaid involves a detailed and often complex process. Applicants must gather necessary documentation, complete various forms, and provide comprehensive financial information to the Medicaid agency. Assistance from Medicaid specialists, social workers, or elder law attorneys can be critical in navigating this process smoothly. These professionals can help address challenges, answer questions, and ensure that the application accurately reflects the applicant's financial situation and care needs.

Medicaid Coverage for Alzheimer's Care: Medicaid covers a broad spectrum of services for individuals with Alzheimer's disease, including home and community-based services (HCBS), nursing home care, and specialized dementia care programs. Many states offer Medicaid waivers that allow recipients to receive care in their homes or communities rather than in institutional settings. Understanding the services covered and how to access them through Medicaid waivers or other programs is crucial for ensuring that individuals with Alzheimer's receive appropriate care in the least restrictive environment possible.

Medicaid serves as a critical resource for individuals with Alzheimer's disease, offering a way to access necessary long-term care services when private funds are insufficient. By carefully navigating Medicaid's eligibility criteria, employing strategic planning, and understanding the covered services, individuals and families can secure essential care while mitigating financial impact. Incorporating Medicaid planning into a comprehensive care strategy is critical to managing the challenges of Alzheimer's disease and ensuring access to quality care and support services.

Financial Planning in the United Kingdom

Budgeting for Care

Budgeting for Alzheimer's disease in the United Kingdom requires a comprehensive approach to managing immediate and long-term financial challenges. This process involves carefully assessing care costs, maximizing public services, seeking financial assistance, and planning for future needs. Here's a closer look at these critical aspects:

Assessing Care Costs: The first step in budgeting for Alzheimer's care is to evaluate the current and anticipated costs associated with the disease. This includes the costs of residential care or nursing homes for those who require full-time care, home care services for assistance with daily activities, medications, and any necessary adaptations to the home to ensure safety and accessibility. Additional costs might include support services like day centers, which provide social opportunities and respite for caregivers or professional respite care services to allow caregivers short breaks from their duties.

Utilizing Public Services: The National Health Service (NHS) and local authorities in the UK offer various services that can help manage care costs. NHS-funded continuing healthcare is a significant support for those with complex medical needs, covering the total cost of care for eligible individuals. Additionally, social care assessments provided by local authorities can identify needs and recommend services, some of which may be funded or subsidized, depending on the individual's financial situation.

Seeking Financial Assistance: Financial assistance is available through means-tested benefits designed to support individuals with disabilities and their caregivers. Attendance Allowance, Disability Living Allowance (DLA), Personal Independence Payment (PIP), and Carer's Allowance are vital benefits that can help offset care costs. These benefits are based on the level of need rather than income, although there are financial assessments for some of these supports to determine eligibility.

Planning for Future Needs: Looking ahead is crucial in managing Alzheimer's care. As the condition progresses, care needs can increase, potentially leading to higher costs. Planning for these eventualities involves setting aside funds through savings or investments and considering options for long-term care insurance, which can provide additional financial resources when more intensive care is needed. It's also essential to explore legal and financial planning tools, such as lasting power of attorney, to ensure decisions regarding care and finances can be made in the best interest of the individual with Alzheimer's.

By addressing these aspects of budgeting for care, individuals and families can create a more secure financial foundation to navigate the complexities of Alzheimer's disease and dementia care. This proactive approach allows for better management of the disease's financial impact, ensuring that individuals with Alzheimer's can access the care and support they need throughout their journey.

Long-Term Care Insurance

Long-term care insurance in the United Kingdom allows individuals to supplement their care provision, providing additional financial protection and peace of mind. While not as prevalent as in some other countries, there are still viable options for those looking to secure their future care needs. Here are some considerations for individuals exploring long-term care insurance in the UK:

Private Insurance Policies: Various insurance companies and specialist providers offer private long-term care insurance. These policies are designed to cover the costs associated with long-term care, whether in a residential care home or through home care services. The specific terms, coverage limits, and types of care covered can vary significantly between policies, so it's important to carefully review these details to find a policy that meets your needs.

Policy Features and Limitations: Understanding the features and limitations of long-term care insurance policies is crucial. This includes clarifying the eligibility criteria, such as age and health status at the time of application; benefit amounts, which determine how much the policy will pay out for care costs; waiting periods before benefits start; and any exclusions, particularly for pre-existing conditions. These factors can significantly affect the usefulness and effectiveness of a policy in meeting your care needs.

Affordability and Accessibility: The cost of long-term care insurance premiums can vary widely based on factors such as the individual's age, health status, and the level of coverage desired. Given your financial resources, assessing whether the premiums are affordable and sustainable over the long term is essential. Consulting with independent financial advisors can be beneficial in comparing policy options, understanding the nuances of each policy, and making an informed decision that aligns with your financial situation and care planning goals.

Integration with Public Services: When considering long-term care insurance, it's also wise to consider how it can complement existing public services. The UK offers care funding and support through the NHS and local authorities. Understanding how long-term care insurance can fill gaps in public provision can help create a more comprehensive and cohesive plan for financing care needs. This might involve using insurance to cover costs not met by public funding or to enhance the quality and choice of care available.

While long-term care insurance might not be the right solution for everyone, it can provide additional financial security for those who choose to explore it. It enables individuals to maintain greater control over their care arrangements and ensures they can access the care they desire without relying solely on public funding options. As with any significant financial decision, it's essential to conduct thorough research, seek expert advice, and consider how insurance fits into broader financial and care planning strategies.

Public Funding and Assistance

In the United Kingdom, navigating the landscape of care for individuals with Alzheimer's disease involves understanding the various sources of public funding and assistance available. These resources are crucial for providing comprehensive support and care to those affected by these conditions and their caregivers. Here's a closer look at the critical aspects of public funding and assistance:

NHS Continuing Healthcare is a vital component of the support system. It offers a fully funded care package for individuals with complex medical needs, such as those in advanced stages of Alzheimer's who require continuous healthcare. A multidisciplinary team thoroughly assesses the nature, complexity, intensity, and unpredictability of the individual's needs. If eligible, this package covers the total cost of care, including accommodation and healthcare needs, in various settings.

Local Authority Support plays a significant role in providing care and assistance. Local authorities are responsible for conducting social care assessments for individuals with Alzheimer's to identify their needs and determine the most appropriate forms of support. This can include in-home care services, day center placements, and residential care. Financial assistance from local authorities is means-tested, meaning it considers the individual's income and savings to determine eligibility for support. For those with limited financial resources, this can significantly reduce the burden of care costs.

Means-tested benefits are designed to provide financial aid to individuals with Alzheimer's and their caregivers. Benefits such as the Attendance Allowance, Disability Living Allowance (DLA), Personal Independence Payment (PIP), and Carer's Allowance are available depending on the individual's circumstances and level of need. These benefits are intended to help cover the additional costs associated with long-term care and support, making them an essential component of financial planning for families affected by Alzheimer's.

Planning for Eligibility is a crucial step in accessing public funding and assistance. Families and individuals are encouraged to plan for the assessment and means-testing process. This involves gathering the necessary documentation, understanding the criteria for different types of support, and seeking advice from local authorities or independent advisors. Planning can help maximize entitlements to public funding and assistance, ensuring that individuals with Alzheimer's and their caregivers receive the support they need.

Incorporating information about these public funding and assistance programs into comprehensive care planning is essential for managing the financial challenges of Alzheimer's disease and dementia care in the UK. By leveraging these resources, individuals and families can ensure access to necessary care and support services, alleviating some of the financial pressures associated with long-term care and enabling a focus on quality of life and well-being for those affected by Alzheimer's.

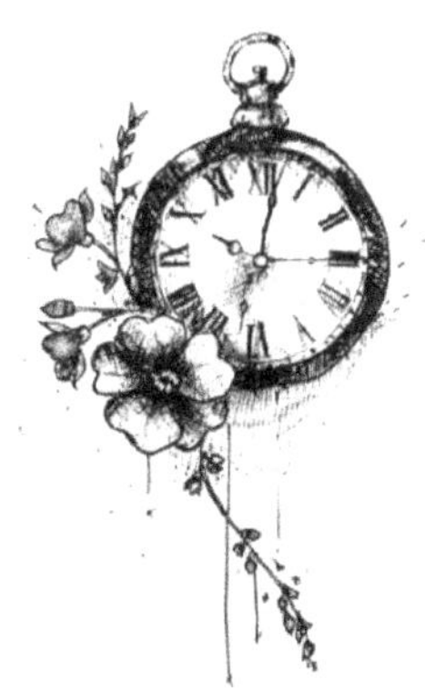

Chapter Seven – Caring for Yourself as a Caregiver

Understanding Caregiver Stress

Caring for a loved one with Alzheimer's disease can be both rewarding and challenging. In this section, we'll explore the concept of caregiver stress, its effects, and coping strategies.

What is Caregiver Stress?

Caregiver stress, also known as caregiver burden or caregiver burnout, refers to the physical, emotional, and psychological strain experienced by individuals who provide care and support to a loved one with Alzheimer's disease. Caregiver stress can manifest in various ways and may be influenced by factors such as the severity of the loved one's condition, the duration of caregiving responsibilities, and the availability of support resources.

The Effects of Caregiver Stress

Caregiver stress, stemming from the continuous demands of caring for someone with Alzheimer's disease, can manifest in several detrimental ways, affecting both the caregiver and the quality of care provided. Understanding these impacts is essential for recognizing the need for support and implementing strategies to mitigate stress.

Physical Health Impacts: The physical toll on caregivers can be significant. Chronic stress can lead to a host of physical health problems, including fatigue, sleep disturbances, headaches, and digestive issues. This is often the result of putting the care recipient's needs before their own, leading to neglect of their health and well-being. Also, constant stress can weaken the immune system, making caregivers more susceptible to illnesses. These physical manifestations affect the caregiver's health and can compromise their ability to provide care.

Emotional and Psychological Strain: The emotional and psychological challenges caregivers face can be overwhelming. Anxiety and depression are common, fueled by the demanding nature of caregiving and the emotional pain of watching a loved one decline. Feelings of guilt or resentment may arise, especially if the caregiver feels trapped in their role or believes they're not doing enough for their loved one. Social isolation can exacerbate these feelings, as caregivers might withdraw from social activities and support networks due to their caregiving responsibilities, leading to decreased self-esteem and a sense of loneliness.

Relationship Strain: The stress of caregiving can also strain relationships with family members, friends, and the care recipient.

Conflicts and misunderstandings may become more frequent as the caregiver's time and emotional capacity are stretched thin. Frustration or resentment can emerge, particularly if the caregiver feels unsupported by other family members or if the caregiving responsibilities disrupt personal relationships. This strain can negatively affect the caregiver's social support network, which is crucial for their well-being.

Decreased Quality of Care: Perhaps one of the most concerning effects of caregiver stress is the potential decrease in the quality of care provided to the individual with Alzheimer's disease. Stress can lead to lapses in attention and judgment, making it more challenging to manage the complex needs of the care recipient. There's also an increased risk of neglecting the care recipient's basic needs due to being overwhelmed or burnt out. This affects the caregiver's sense of competency and satisfaction and directly impacts the health and happiness of the person they are caring for.

These effects underscore the importance of addressing caregiver stress through supportive measures, such as seeking help from support groups, utilizing respite care services, prioritizing self-care, and setting realistic expectations for caregiving. By acknowledging and managing the impacts of caregiver stress, caregivers can protect their well-being and ensure they provide the best possible care to their loved ones.

Coping with Caregiver Stress

Coping with caregiver stress is a critical aspect of providing care for a loved one with Alzheimer's disease. The responsibility of caregiving, while deeply rewarding, can also be incredibly challenging, leading to high levels of stress that affect both the caregiver's and the recipient's quality of life. Implementing effective coping strategies is essential for maintaining the well-being of both parties. Here's how caregivers can manage and alleviate stress:

Seek support, which is the first step in managing caregiver stress. Building a network of support is vital. This can include family members, friends, support groups, or professional caregivers. Emotional support from those who understand your challenges can provide significant relief. Practical assistance with caregiving duties can help lighten the load, and respite care can offer a much-needed break. Support groups, whether in person or online, can also provide a sense of community and shared invaluable understanding.

Prioritize Self-Care is fundamental for coping with caregiver stress. Engaging in self-care activities such as regular exercise, relaxation techniques like meditation or yoga, healthy eating, ensuring adequate sleep, and enjoying leisure activities can significantly impact physical and emotional well-being. These activities help prevent caregiver burnout by replenishing your energy and reducing stress levels, enabling you to continue providing care with patience and compassion.

Set Realistic Expectations for yourself and the caregiving situation. It is understanding that you're doing your best in a challenging situation. Recognize the limits of what you can provide and know that it's okay to ask for help. Setting realistic expectations helps manage the pressures of caregiving, reduce feelings of guilt or inadequacy, and prioritize tasks most critical to your loved one's care.

Utilize Respite Care Services to take a step back and recharge. Respite care, offered by community organizations, adult day centers, or professional caregivers, can provide temporary relief from caregiving responsibilities. This break is essential for your well-being, allowing you time to rest, pursue personal interests, or relax, which is crucial for maintaining your health and stamina for caregiving.

Educate Yourself about Alzheimer's disease. Gaining knowledge about the disease, caregiving techniques, and the resources available can empower you as a caregiver. Education can help you feel more in control and reduce anxiety by helping you understand what to expect and how to respond to various situations. Knowledge about support services can also connect you to additional resources to ease the caregiving journey.

Understanding caregiver stress and implementing these coping strategies can significantly improve the caregiving experience. By prioritizing your health and well-being, you're taking care of yourself and enhancing the care you can provide your loved one. Remember, caring for yourself is essential to being a caregiver. It's not selfish; it's necessary to provide the best possible care to your loved one with Alzheimer's disease.

Self-Care for Caregivers

Caring for a loved one with Alzheimer's disease can be emotionally and physically demanding. In this section, we'll explore the importance of self-care for caregivers and provide strategies for maintaining well-being while navigating the challenges of caregiving.

The Importance of Self-Care for Caregivers

Self-care is not just a concept but a crucial practice for caregivers tending to loved ones with Alzheimer's disease. It embodies a comprehensive approach to maintaining one's health, emotional resilience, and overall well-being, enabling caregivers to navigate the complexities of their roles with strength and compassion. The significance of self-care for caregivers extends across several dimensions:

Preservation of Health is paramount. Caregivers often experience continuous stress, which can affect their physical health. It is vital to prioritize self-care activities such as regular exercise, nutritious eating, ensuring adequate sleep, and adopting stress management techniques. These practices help maintain physical health, boost immune function, and reduce the risk of chronic stress and fatigue exacerbations. Moreover, they play a critical role in preventing caregiver burnout, a state of physical, emotional, and mental exhaustion that can dramatically affect one's ability to provide care.

Emotional Resilience is fortified through self-care. The emotional demands of caregiving—witnessing the decline of a loved one, managing daily challenges, and navigating the complexities of care—can evoke feelings of anxiety, sadness, and isolation. Caregivers can alleviate stress and foster a sense of well-being by engaging in self-care activities such as relaxation techniques, pursuing hobbies, and socializing. These practices enable caregivers to build emotional resilience, equipping them to handle the ups and downs of caregiving with more excellent stability and strength.

Enhanced Caregiving Abilities result from a well-cared-for caregiver. Self-care is not an act of selfishness but a necessity for those providing care. When caregivers take time to care for themselves, they recharge their batteries, enhancing their capacity to offer compassionate, patient, and attentive care to their loved ones. A caregiver who is physically healthy, emotionally stable, and psychologically resilient is better equipped to meet the demands of caregiving, respond to the needs of their loved one with Alzheimer's, and navigate the challenges that arise with patience and understanding.

Improved Quality of Life is a significant outcome of consistent self-care. Caregiving can consume a caregiver's life, leaving little room for personal growth, relaxation, and fulfillment outside their caregiving responsibilities. Investing in self-care helps caregivers maintain balance and personal fulfillment, contributing to a better quality of life. It allows them to enjoy moments of joy, pursue interests, and maintain relationships, fostering a sense of identity beyond their caregiving role. This balance is essential for sustaining the caregiver's happiness, satisfaction, and overall quality of life amidst the demands of caregiving.

Strategies for Self-Care

The importance of self-care cannot be overstated in the challenging journey of caring for individuals with Alzheimer's. Caregivers often put their needs on the back burner, focusing all their energy and attention on the person they care for. However, neglecting self-care can lead to burnout, reduced health, and diminished capacity to provide care. Effective self-care strategies are crucial for maintaining the caregiver's physical, emotional, and mental well-being.

Establishing Boundaries is a fundamental self-care strategy. It involves defining clear limits around caregiving responsibilities, personal time, and social commitments. By setting these boundaries, caregivers can protect their well-being and ensure they have enough energy and resources to care for their loved ones effectively. Balancing caregiving duties and personal life helps manage stress and prevent caregiver fatigue.

Mindfulness and Relaxation techniques, such as mindfulness meditation, deep breathing exercises, yoga, or other relaxation methods, can significantly reduce stress and promote emotional well-being. These practices help center the mind, calm the body, and reduce the physiological symptoms of stress. Incorporating these techniques into the daily routine can provide caregivers with a much-needed mental break and help maintain a sense of peace amidst the challenges of caregiving.

Another vital self-care strategy is engaging in **Hobbies and Interests** that bring joy and relaxation. Caregivers should make time for gardening, reading, painting, or listening to music. These hobbies can serve as a therapeutic escape from the demands of caregiving, offering a sense of normalcy and personal fulfillment. They provide an essential outlet for stress and can rejuvenate the caregiver's spirit.

Seeking Social Support from friends, family, support groups, or online communities dedicated to caregiving can offer a lifeline to caregivers. Sharing experiences, seeking advice, and receiving emotional support from others who understand the unique challenges of caregiving can provide a sense of community and belonging. This social support is invaluable for combating feelings of isolation and provides caregivers with a network of individuals who can offer practical advice and emotional solace.

Taking Breaks from caregiving duties is essential to avoid burnout. Regularly scheduled breaks allow caregivers to rest, recharge, and engage in activities unrelated to caregiving. Utilizing respite care services or enlisting the help of family members or professional caregivers can provide relief and ensure caregivers can take these important breaks. These rest periods are crucial for maintaining the caregiver's health and well-being, allowing them to continue providing high-quality care.

Finding Support

Finding support as a caregiver is essential for managing the demands of caregiving and maintaining well-being. Ways to find support include:

Joining Support Groups: Support groups provide a platform for caregivers of individuals with Alzheimer's to meet, share experiences, and exchange coping strategies. These groups, available in person and online, offer a sense of community and understanding, making caregivers feel less isolated. Participants can learn from others' experiences, gaining insights into managing daily challenges, navigating healthcare systems, and maintaining emotional health. Many find solace and practical advice in these gatherings, enhancing their ability to care for their loved ones while looking after their well-being.

Seeking Professional Help: In the journey of caregiving for someone with Alzheimer's, the emotional and psychological toll on the caregiver can be profound. The responsibilities are not just physically demanding but also emotionally draining, leading to feelings of stress, anxiety, depression, and what is often termed caregiver burnout. These emotional challenges can significantly impact a caregiver's quality of life, affecting their ability to provide care. Recognizing and addressing these feelings is a crucial aspect of self-care that cannot be overlooked.

Seeking professional help from a mental health professional, such as a psychologist or a counselor, is a valuable step for caregivers who find themselves struggling with these emotional burdens. These professionals can offer a supportive space for caregivers to express their feelings, concerns, and frustrations without judgment. Through counseling or therapy, caregivers can learn coping strategies to manage stress, anxiety, and depression, helping them navigate their emotions more effectively.

Professional support can also provide caregivers with tools and techniques to recognize the signs of burnout early on and take proactive steps to mitigate its effects. Burnout can manifest in various ways, including physical exhaustion, irritability, changes in sleep patterns, feelings of hopelessness, and a detachment from the caregiving role. A mental health professional can help caregivers develop personalized strategies for self-care, set healthy boundaries, and find a balance between caregiving responsibilities and personal needs.

Moreover, therapy can facilitate the exploration of complex emotions related to caregiving, such as guilt, grief, and anger. These feelings are common among caregivers but are often suppressed due to societal expectations or personal beliefs about duty and family roles. A therapist can help unpack these emotions, providing a path toward understanding and acceptance.

Utilizing Respite Care Services: These services are vital as they offer caregivers a necessary break, helping them avoid burnout and maintain their well-being.

Respite care can be found through various sources, including community organizations, adult day centers, and professional caregiving services. These providers offer temporary care that allows primary caregivers some time off from their caregiving duties. This can range from a few hours to several days, depending on the caregiver's needs and the availability of services. During this time, individuals with Alzheimer's can engage in different activities, socialize, and receive professional care tailored to their needs, which can be particularly beneficial for their overall well-being and provide a stimulating environment that might not always be possible at home.

Engaging with respite care services not only supports the physical health of the person with Alzheimer's by ensuring trained professionals look after them but also addresses the emotional and psychological needs of the caregivers. Caregiving for someone with Alzheimer's can be a 24/7 responsibility that can quickly become overwhelming, leading to stress, depression, and physical health issues among caregivers. By taking advantage of respite care, caregivers can take necessary breaks, whether it's to run errands, spend time with other family members, rest, or pursue personal interests. This helps maintain a balance in their lives, reduces stress, and allows them to continue providing care over the long term without sacrificing their health and happiness.

Incorporating the importance and benefits of respite care services into your book will provide caregivers with valuable information and emphasize the community and professional support available to them. Highlighting these services underscores the message that taking care of oneself is not a luxury but a necessity for caregivers, enabling them to be more effective and compassionate.

Communicating Needs: Effective communication is a cornerstone for managing the multifaceted challenges in Alzheimer's caregiving. Caregivers often bear a heavy burden, juggling caregiving's emotional, physical, and logistical aspects. They need to articulate their needs and limitations to family members, friends, and healthcare providers, ensuring a support network that can rally around them when assistance is needed.

Communicating needs involves more than just asking for help; it's about expressing how support is required, whether for physical tasks, emotional support, or simply needing time for oneself. It means being open about what you can and cannot handle and setting realistic expectations for yourself and others. This transparency helps prevent misunderstandings and ensures the caregiver's well-being is prioritized, fostering a healthier caregiving environment.

Many caregivers hesitate to ask for help, driven by feelings of obligation, guilt, or the fear of imposing on others. However, it's essential to recognize that caregiving is not a journey alone. By clearly communicating needs, caregivers can distribute the responsibilities, alleviate stress, and reduce the risk of burnout. Friends and family often want to help but may not know how or what is needed. Providing them with specific tasks or roles can make it easier for them to provide meaningful support.

Healthcare providers also play a critical role in the caregiving ecosystem. They can offer resources, support, and advice on managing the complexities of Alzheimer's care. Communicating openly with these professionals about the caregiver's emotional state and the challenges faced at home and seeking guidance on care strategies can enhance the quality of care provided to the person with Alzheimer's. It also ensures that caregivers can access professional advice and support tailored to their unique circumstances.

By prioritizing self-care, implementing effective coping strategies, and seeking support from others, caregivers can better navigate the demands of caring for a loved one with Alzheimer's disease while safeguarding their well-being and quality of life. Remember, taking care of yourself is not selfish – providing the best care possible to your loved one is necessary.

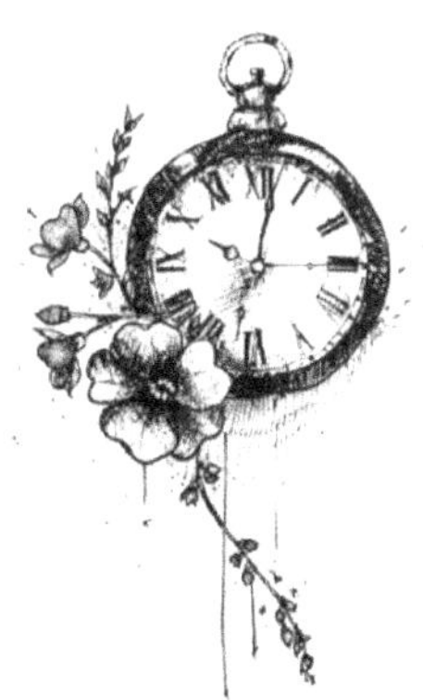

Chapter Eight – Resources for Caregivers

Understanding Available Resources

Accessing support and resources is crucial for caregivers of loved ones with Alzheimer's disease. In this section, we'll explore the types of resources available to caregivers, how to find them in your area, and how to evaluate their suitability for your needs.

Types of Resources Available to Caregivers

Understanding and accessing the array of resources available can significantly alleviate the burden on caregivers of individuals with Alzheimer's disease. Let's delve into how these resources can support caregivers in their journey:

Support Groups: Local support groups allow caregivers to connect with others in similar situations. They serve as a vital source of emotional support and practical advice, offering a platform for sharing experiences and strategies for coping with the challenges of caregiving.

Support groups can be found through local Alzheimer's associations, hospitals, community centers, or online platforms dedicated to caregiver support.

Educational Programs: These programs are designed to provide caregivers with crucial information on Alzheimer's disease, including caregiving techniques, effective communication strategies, and ways to manage behavioral symptoms. Educational resources can be accessed through Alzheimer's associations, healthcare institutions, and community organizations, often offering both in-person and online learning opportunities.

Respite Care Services: Respite care is an essential service that offers caregivers a much-needed break and ensures their loved one is cared for in their absence. This temporary relief can be found through home health agencies, adult day care centers, or community-based services, allowing caregivers time to rest, attend to personal matters, or engage in self-care activities.

Caregiver Training and Workshops: These programs equip caregivers with practical skills and strategies to manage their caregiving responsibilities effectively. They cover topics such as handling challenging behaviors and promoting the well-being of both the caregiver and the person with Alzheimer's. These workshops can be sourced from Alzheimer's associations, community health organizations, and online caregiving resources.

Counseling and Therapy: Access to counseling and therapy services is crucial for caregivers coping with the emotional toll of caregiving. These services provide a safe space to discuss feelings, develop coping strategies, and learn stress management techniques. Therapists specializing in caregiver support can be found through healthcare providers, mental health clinics, and caregiver support organizations.

Financial and Legal Assistance: Navigating caregiving's financial and legal aspects can be daunting. Assistance in this area can include guidance on financial planning, understanding insurance and benefits, and preparing legal documents like powers of attorney and advance directives. Resources for financial and legal assistance can be accessed through elder law attorneys, financial planning services specializing in eldercare, and community legal aid societies.

Evaluating the suitability of these resources involves considering the specific needs of the caregiver and the person with Alzheimer's and the quality, accessibility, and affordability of the services offered. By leveraging these resources, caregivers can enhance their ability to provide care, reduce stress, and improve their overall quality of life and that of their loved ones.

How to Find Resources in Your Area

Finding resources in your area that cater to the needs of caregivers for individuals with Alzheimer's disease can be instrumental in navigating the caregiving journey more effectively. Here's a step-by-step guide on how to locate these vital resources:

Contact Local Alzheimer's Organizations: Contact local branches of national Alzheimer's organizations, such as the Alzheimer's Association or Alzheimer's Society. These organizations often have comprehensive lists of support groups, educational programs, and other specialized caregiver services. They can provide information on resources specific to your community, including contact details and how to access these services.

Consult Healthcare Providers: Your loved one's healthcare team can be a valuable resource for local support and service recommendations. Doctors, nurses, and social workers familiar with your loved one's case may have insights into the most appropriate resources to aid in caregiving. They can suggest respite care options, therapist or counselor contacts specializing in caregiver support, and workshops or training programs for caregivers.

Search Online Directories: The Internet hosts a wealth of directories and databases dedicated to caregiver support services. These online platforms allow you to search for resources based on your geographic location, the type of support you're seeking, and your loved one's specific needs. Websites of national Alzheimer's organizations, healthcare institutions, and caregiver support networks often feature searchable directories to help you find local respite care providers, support groups, and educational resources.

Attend Community Events: Participating in community events such as health fairs, caregiver conferences, and workshops can provide direct access to a wide range of resources. These events often feature booths or presentations from local service providers, support groups, and healthcare professionals. They offer an opportunity to gather information, ask questions, and network with other caregivers and professionals who can guide you toward the necessary resources.

By following these steps, caregivers can access a network of support and resources designed to assist them in providing care, managing stress, and ensuring the well-being of themselves and their loved ones with Alzheimer's disease. Leveraging these resources can significantly improve the caregiving experience, offering practical help, emotional support, and a sense of community among those navigating similar challenges.

Evaluating Resources

Evaluating resources effectively is crucial for caregivers to ensure they find the best support available for both themselves and their loved ones with Alzheimer's disease. Here's a closer look at the key factors to consider when assessing the suitability of caregiving resources:

Relevance to Your Needs: The first step in evaluating a resource is to assess its relevance to your situation. The needs of caregivers and their loved ones can vary greatly, from managing behavioral symptoms and navigating daily care challenges to accessing respite care or obtaining specialized legal and financial advice. Ensure the resource addresses the areas you need support in, whether it's practical caregiving strategies, emotional support, or navigating healthcare systems.

Credibility and Trustworthiness: It's essential to verify the credibility and trustworthiness of the organization or service provider offering the resource. Look for resources provided by reputable nonprofit organizations, government agencies, accredited healthcare institutions, or well-regarded service providers. Research their history, mission, and the populations they serve. Reading reviews and seeking recommendations from healthcare professionals or fellow caregivers can also provide insights into the resource's reliability.

Accessibility and Affordability: Accessibility is a critical factor, encompassing not only the physical location of services but also their availability through online platforms, the flexibility of hours of operation, and any language or communication support offered. Additionally, consider the affordability of the resource, including any costs or fees associated with accessing the service, eligibility criteria for financial assistance, or sliding scale fees to ensure the resource is financially viable for your situation.

Quality of Services: Evaluating the quality of services involves examining the qualifications and experience of the staff or volunteers, the comprehensiveness of the services provided, and the overall approach to care and support. Feedback from other caregivers who have utilized the resource can be invaluable, providing real-world insights into what to expect and the service's benefits. Online reviews, testimonials, and caregiver forums can help gather this information.

By thoroughly considering these factors, caregivers can make informed decisions about the resources they pursue, ensuring they receive the support and assistance needed to manage the complexities of caregiving for someone with Alzheimer's. Remember, finding the right resources can significantly impact the caregiving experience, offering crucial support, enhancing the quality of care, and improving the well-being of the caregiver and their loved one.

Support Groups for Caregivers

Support groups are a vital resource for caregivers of individuals with Alzheimer's disease. In this section, we'll explore the benefits of support groups, the various types available, and how caregivers can find a support group that meets their needs.

The Benefits of Support Groups for Caregivers

Support groups play a crucial role in the well-being of caregivers, offering a wide range of benefits that can significantly enhance their ability to provide care while maintaining their health and emotional resilience. Here are some of the critical advantages of participating in a support group:

Emotional Support: One of the primary benefits of support groups is their emotional support. Caregivers can connect with others facing similar challenges, creating a sense of community and belonging. This connection provides validation and empathy, allowing caregivers to feel understood and less isolated in their experiences.

Information and Education: Support groups often serve as a valuable resource for information and education on various aspects of caregiving. They may offer access to expert speakers, literature, and resources that can help caregivers better understand Alzheimer's, effective caregiving techniques, and the support services available. This knowledge can empower caregivers, equipping them with the tools they need to provide the best care for their loved ones.

Coping Strategies: Through sharing experiences and advice, caregivers can learn new coping strategies from their peers in the group. These strategies can help manage stress, handle difficult emotions, and navigate the complexities of caregiving. Learning from others who have faced similar situations can provide practical tips and innovative solutions to common caregiving challenges.

Peer Validation: Support groups offer a safe space for caregivers to share their experiences and express their feelings openly. Receiving validation and understanding from others in similar situations can be incredibly affirming, helping caregivers recognize the value of their efforts and the commonality of their experiences.

Problem-Solving: A support group's collective wisdom provides a rich resource for problem-solving. Caregivers can discuss specific issues, brainstorm solutions, and offer each other practical advice. This collaborative approach can lead to effective strategies for overcoming challenges and making caregiving tasks more manageable.

Overall, the benefits of support groups for caregivers extend far beyond these key areas, offering a lifeline to those who dedicate their lives to caring for others. By participating in a support group, caregivers can find the strength, knowledge, and support they need to continue their caregiving journey with confidence and compassion.

Types of Support Groups Available to Caregivers

Caregivers can access various support groups designed to meet different needs and preferences. Understanding the types of support groups available can help caregivers choose the one that best suits their situation:

In-Person Support Groups: These groups offer face-to-face meetings in community settings such as hospitals, senior centers, or religious institutions. They allow caregivers to connect directly with others in their area who are going through similar experiences. Other members' physical presence can provide camaraderie and immediate emotional support, making these groups particularly valuable for those who benefit from direct interaction.

Online Support Groups: For caregivers who may face time constraints or geographical limitations or prefer the anonymity of the internet, online support groups offer a flexible alternative. These groups can be forums, social media communities, or video conference meetings, allowing caregivers to share experiences, advice, and support with others from the comfort of their homes at any time of day.

Disease-Specific Support Groups: Focusing on specific conditions, such as Alzheimer's disease, these support groups provide specialized information, resources, and support. They cater to the unique challenges faced by caregivers of individuals with these conditions, offering insights into disease management, coping strategies, and the latest research findings. Joining a disease-specific support group can be incredibly helpful for those seeking advice and support tailored to their loved one's condition.

Caregiver-Specific Support Groups: These groups are designed to support caregivers regardless of the specific condition their loved one is facing. They focus on the universal aspects of caregiving, offering education, resources, and emotional support to individuals caring for loved ones with various health issues. Caregiver-specific support groups can provide valuable coping strategies, stress management techniques, and a broader perspective on the caregiving experience.

Choosing the right type of support group depends on the caregiver's specific needs, preferences, and the nature of their caregiving situation. Each type of group offers unique benefits, and caregivers may find it helpful to explore multiple options to find the best fit for their needs. Engaging with a support group can significantly impact a caregiver's emotional well-being, providing a sense of understanding, community, and shared experience vital for navigating the caregiving journey.

Finding a Support Group

Finding a support group can be a lifeline for caregivers navigating the complexities of caring for someone with Alzheimer's or another form of dementia. Here are steps to help locate a support group that fits your needs:

Contact Local Organizations: Contact local Alzheimer's associations, caregiver support organizations, hospitals, and community centers. These institutions often have up-to-date information on support groups in your area and can direct you to resources that match your specific situation.

Search Online: Utilize online directories and resources from national organizations, such as the Alzheimer's Association or healthcare providers. These platforms allow you to search for support groups based on your location, the type of support you seek, or specific needs related to the care recipient's condition.

Attend Events: Participate in caregiver conferences, health fairs, or community events. Such gatherings often have information booths or representatives from various support groups. These events provide an excellent opportunity to learn more about available support, ask questions, and meet group organizers or members in person.

Ask for Recommendations: Don't hesitate to ask healthcare providers, social workers, friends, or family members for recommendations. Often, personal referrals can lead you to the most supportive and relevant groups. Those who have had direct experience with support groups can provide insights into the benefits and atmosphere of different groups, helping you make an informed decision.

Participating in a support group allows caregivers to connect with others who genuinely understand caregiving's emotional and physical challenges. These groups provide a safe space to share experiences, access valuable information and resources, and find comfort in the solidarity of others facing similar situations. Remember, seeking support is a sign of strength and an essential step in maintaining your well-being while caring for a loved one.

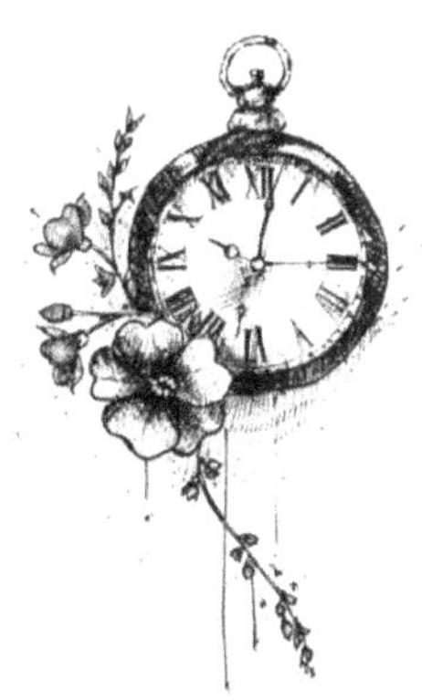

Chapter Nine: Understanding End-of-Life Care

What is End-of-Life Care?

End-of-life care encompasses a range of supportive services and interventions provided to individuals with advanced Alzheimer's disease. It focuses on meeting their physical, emotional, and spiritual needs as they near the end of their lives. End-of-life care aims to ensure comfort, alleviate distressing symptoms, promote dignity, and enhance the overall quality of life during the terminal phase of the disease.

Critical components of end-of-life care may include pain management, symptom control, assistance with activities of daily living, emotional and psychological support for both the individual and their family members, spiritual care, and assistance with advance care planning and decision-making.

Depending on the individual's preferences, care needs, and available resources, end-of-life care may be provided in various settings, including home-based care, hospice care facilities, nursing homes, or hospitals.

The Importance of End-of-Life Care

End-of-life care is essential for ensuring that individuals with Alzheimer's disease receive compassionate and appropriate care that honors their preferences, values, and wishes as they approach the end of their lives. The importance of end-of-life care includes:

Ensuring Comfort and Quality of Life: This aspect of end-of-life care is about more than just managing physical symptoms; it's about enhancing the overall quality of life for those in their final stages of Alzheimer's. Techniques include medical pain and symptom relief interventions and environmental adjustments to create a calming, familiar setting. Tailoring activities that the individual can enjoy or find comfort in, such as listening to favorite music or having family photos nearby, contributes to their dignity and comfort.

Respecting Autonomy and Choices: At the heart of respecting autonomy is the principle that individuals should have the right to choose their end-of-life care based on their values and preferences. This process often involves detailed discussions with healthcare providers to understand the implications of different care options and use advance directives to document those choices. It's about ensuring that the individual's voice is heard and respected, even when they can no longer communicate their wishes directly.

Providing Emotional and Spiritual Support: Emotional and spiritual support is tailored to meet the individual needs of the person and their family, recognizing that each person's journey is unique. Support may include counseling services to help navigate the grief process, spiritual care that aligns with the individual's beliefs, and creating opportunities for meaningful interactions with loved ones. This holistic approach acknowledges the complex emotions involved in end-of-life care and offers a compassionate presence to those navigating this challenging time.

Facilitating Meaningful Endings: Facilitating meaningful endings involves creating opportunities for individuals and their families to engage in activities that promote closure and peace. This might include helping the individual to record messages for loved ones, arranging visits or video calls with distant family members, or organizing small, intimate gatherings that honor the individual's life and legacy. These actions help ensure that the end-of-life phase is marked by moments of connection, reflection, and dignity, honoring the individual's journey and impact on those around them.

Each of these components is critical to providing end-of-life care that is compassionate, respectful, and aligned with the individual's wishes, offering a pathway to peace and dignity in the final days.

How to Prepare for End-of-Life Care

Caregivers can prepare for end-of-life care by taking the following steps:

Having Conversations About End-of-Life Wishes: Discussing end-of-life preferences is essential for understanding the individual's wishes regarding their care. These conversations should cover various topics, including preferences for medical interventions, hospice care, and the individual's feelings about life-sustaining treatments. It's essential to approach these discussions with sensitivity, allowing the person to express their desires freely and ensuring that their wishes are documented and understood by all involved in their care.

Completing Advance Care Planning Documents: Advance care planning involves preparing legal documents that outline the individual's healthcare preferences. These documents, such as living wills and durable powers of attorney for healthcare, ensure that the person's medical wishes are respected, especially in situations where they might not be able to communicate their decisions. Assistance in completing these documents often involves discussions with healthcare professionals, legal advisors, and family members to ensure that all legal requirements are met and that the documents accurately reflect the individual's wishes.

Identifying and Communicating Care Preferences: This step involves a detailed discussion about the individual's preferences for their end-of-life care, including where they wish to receive care (at home, in a hospice facility, etc.), specific treatment preferences, and how they wish to manage pain and other symptoms. Communicating these preferences to healthcare providers and family members ensures that the care plan is consistent with the individual's values and desires, promoting a more personalized and respectful end-of-life experience.

Establishing a Supportive Care Team: A multidisciplinary team that includes doctors, nurses, social workers, spiritual advisors, and hospice care providers can offer comprehensive support tailored to the individual's needs. This team works collaboratively to provide symptom management, emotional support, and spiritual care according to the individual's wishes. Building this team early ensures a coordinated approach to care encompassing all aspects of the individual's well-being.

Seeking Emotional and Practical Support: Navigating the end-of-life process can be emotionally taxing for the individual and their caregivers. Seeking support from various sources, including family members, friends, professional caregivers, and support groups, can provide the emotional and practical assistance needed during this time. Emotional support can help caregivers and family members cope with their feelings of grief and loss. In contrast, practical support can assist with the daily caregiving tasks, allowing for more quality time spent with the loved one.

By thoroughly addressing these areas, caregivers can ensure that the end-of-life care provided to individuals with Alzheimer's disease is compassionate, respectful, and in line with their wishes, making this challenging time a little easier for everyone involved.

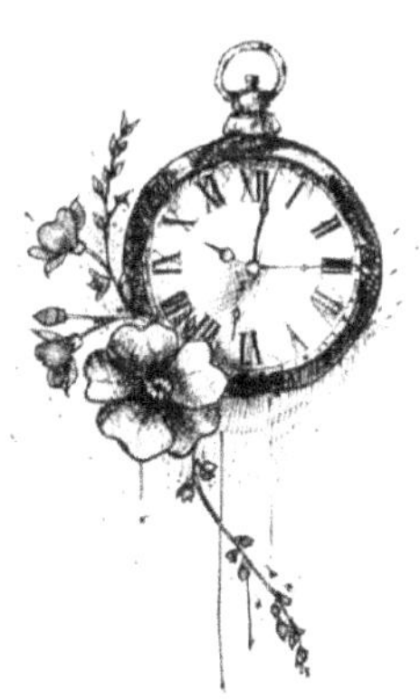

Chapter Ten: Providing End-of-Life Care

End-of-life care is critical to supporting individuals with Alzheimer's disease. It focuses on ensuring comfort, dignity, and quality of life as they approach their final days. This comprehensive care encompasses a wide range of services and approaches, including palliative and hospice care, each tailored to meet the unique needs of the individual and their family during this challenging time.

Palliative care serves as a cornerstone of end-of-life care, relieving the symptoms and stress of a severe illness. Its primary goal is to improve the patient's and their family's quality of life. Unlike hospice care, palliative care is not limited to those nearing the end of life. It can be provided at any stage of a severe illness, including Alzheimer's disease. This holistic care involves a multidisciplinary team that addresses physical symptoms and emotional, social, and spiritual needs. Palliative care supports individuals in navigating the complexities of their illness, offering pain management, symptom control, and assistance in making medical decisions that align with their values and preferences.

Hospice care, on the other hand, is specifically designed for those in the final stages of a life-limiting illness. It represents a shift from curative to comfort-focused care, with the understanding that the focus should be on enhancing the quality of the individual's remaining life rather than attempting to prolong it. This type of care is initiated when it is believed that the individual has six months or less to live if the illness follows its natural course. Hospice care encompasses a broad range of services aimed at managing pain and other symptoms, providing emotional and spiritual support, and offering guidance and counseling to families and caregivers navigating the grieving process. It requires a decision to forgo further curative treatments in favor of treatments aimed at comfort and relief.

In conclusion, end-of-life care for individuals with Alzheimer's disease requires a compassionate, holistic approach that addresses the physical, emotional, and spiritual needs of the individual and their family. Whether through palliative care at any stage of the illness or hospice care in the final months, the focus remains on ensuring comfort, dignity, and quality of life, providing support and guidance as individuals and their loved ones navigate this challenging journey.

Managing Pain and Other Symptoms

Effective management of pain and other symptoms is a cornerstone of providing compassionate and quality end-of-life care for individuals with Alzheimer's disease. These individuals may experience many symptoms that can significantly impact their comfort and quality of life in their final days. Addressing these symptoms with a comprehensive and personalized approach is crucial to ensuring their dignity and comfort.

Pain is a common concern and can often be challenging to assess in individuals with advanced Alzheimer's due to communication difficulties. To manage pain effectively, caregivers and healthcare providers must be attuned to nonverbal cues of discomfort, such as facial expressions, body language, and changes in behavior. Agitation or restlessness, another frequent symptom, can stem from various sources, including physical discomfort, environmental factors, or emotional distress.

Anxiety and depression are also prevalent, affecting individuals' emotional well-being and requiring sensitive intervention. Sleep disturbances, which can exacerbate other symptoms and affect the individual and their caregivers, need tailored approaches to promote restful sleep. Difficulty swallowing and respiratory distress are symptomatic of the disease's progression, necessitating adjustments in care to ensure comfort and prevent complications. Constipation or bowel obstruction and skin breakdown or pressure ulcers indicate the need for diligent physical care and monitoring to maintain the individual's physical well-being.

A multifaceted strategy is employed to manage these diverse symptoms, combining pharmacological and non-pharmacological interventions. Pharmacological interventions, carefully prescribed and monitored by healthcare professionals, include medications for pain relief, anxiety reduction, and sedation to manage specific symptoms effectively. These medications must be used judiciously, considering the individual's condition and potential side effects.

Non-pharmacological approaches play an equally important role in symptom management, offering alternative means of comfort and distress alleviation. Techniques such as massage, music therapy, aromatherapy, and relaxation exercises can provide significant relief and enhance the individual's quality of life. These approaches are particularly valuable as they can be tailored to the individual's preferences and history, offering symptom relief and connecting to personal experiences and memories.

Environmental modifications contribute to symptom management by creating a calm, serene atmosphere that reduces agitation and anxiety. This may involve minimizing noise and other sensory stimuli, ensuring comfortable lighting, and personalizing the space with familiar objects or comforting items that have personal significance to the individual.

Regular assessment and open communication with healthcare providers are essential to managing symptoms effectively. This ongoing dialogue ensures that the care plan remains responsive to the individual's evolving needs, allowing for timely intervention adjustments. It underscores the importance of prioritizing the individual's comfort and well-being throughout illness.

In summary, managing pain and other symptoms in individuals with Alzheimer's disease at the end of life requires a compassionate, holistic approach that integrates pharmacological treatments, non-pharmacological methods, environmental modifications, and proactive communication with healthcare providers. By prioritizing the individual's comfort and dignity, caregivers and healthcare professionals can ensure that the final stage of life is marked by peace and respect.

Coping with Grief and Loss

Coping with grief and loss for caregivers of individuals with Alzheimer's is an intricate, deeply personal journey that unfolds over time, often long before the loss of the loved one in the traditional sense. This grief is multifaceted, encompassing the progressive loss of the person they once knew, even as they physically remain. It demands a compassionate, understanding approach to oneself, recognizing that this form of grieving begins with the diagnosis and continues, evolving as the disease progresses. Each stage brings challenges and requires specific coping mechanisms, from seeking support to acknowledging and expressing the complex emotional tapestry. Caregivers must navigate this path with self-kindness, finding ways to honor their loved one's memory while caring for their emotional well-being. This journey is not linear but a continuous process of adapting, learning, and finding moments of connection and peace amidst the heartache.

Acknowledging and Expressing Emotions

Acknowledging and expressing the range of emotions encountered in the wake of grief and loss is a crucial part of the healing journey for caregivers. This emotional journey often involves navigating through a complex tapestry of feelings such as sadness, anger, guilt, and even relief. These emotions indicate the deep bond and care for the loved one being cared for. Allowing oneself the space and permission to experience and articulate these emotions entirely is essential for healing. Recognizing that these emotional responses are natural and legitimate reactions to the significant changes and losses encountered is essential. By embracing and expressing these feelings, individuals can start to process their grief, facilitating a path toward adjustment and finding peace amidst the profound shifts in their lives. This emotional acknowledgment and expression serve as the bedrock for building resilience and moving forward, grounded in the understanding that these feelings are part of the human experience, especially poignant in the context of caregiving and loss.

Seeking Support

Seeking support in the face of grief and loss is a journey that should never be walked alone. Reaching out to family and friends can offer a foundation of love and understanding, providing comfort during sorrow. Furthermore, support groups bring together individuals who share the common thread of Alzheimer's caregiving, creating a unique community where experiences, challenges, and coping mechanisms can be shared openly. These groups serve as a beacon of hope and understanding, offering solace in the shared journey. Additionally, mental health professionals can provide invaluable guidance, offering therapeutic strategies tailored to navigate the complexities of grief. Through counseling or therapy, individuals can explore their feelings in a safe space, learn healthy coping strategies, and gradually find a path toward healing. This comprehensive support network plays a crucial role in mitigating the overwhelming nature of loss, helping individuals survive and find a way to thrive amidst adversity. Engaging with this support network fosters a sense of belonging, understanding, and hope, which is essential in healing.

Practicing Self-Care

In Alzheimer's care, practicing self-care is not just beneficial; it is necessary to maintain the caregiver's well-being and enhance their ability to provide compassionate support. The journey of caregiving, marked by its emotional highs and lows, demands a deliberate commitment to self-nurturing practices. These practices encompass various activities to rejuvenate the caregiver's physical, emotional, and spiritual health. Regular physical exercise, for instance, can be a powerful antidote to stress, boosting physical stamina and mental clarity. Simultaneously, relaxation techniques such as meditation, deep breathing exercises, or yoga can be vital tools for managing anxiety and fostering a sense of inner peace.

Furthermore, dedicating time to hobbies and interests provides a meaningful escape from the caregiving routine. It allows for personal expression and the pursuit of joy amidst challenging circumstances. These moments of engagement break the monotony and serve as critical outlets for creative and emotional release. Additionally, cultivating connections with friends and family offers emotional sustenance, reminding caregivers that they are not alone in their journey. These relationships can provide a network of support, understanding, and practical assistance when needed.

Self-care also extends to seeking professional support when necessary, whether counseling to navigate personal grief or joining support groups to share experiences and strategies with others in similar situations. These avenues of support can provide validation, encouragement, and a sense of community, which are invaluable during times of caregiving.

Incorporating these self-care practices into daily life requires intentionality and sometimes a shift in perspective. One must recognize that taking care of oneself is not selfish but a crucial component of effective caregiving. It's about finding balance, allowing for moments of respite and self-reflection, which can lead to a more sustainable caregiving experience. By acknowledging the significance of self-care, caregivers can find strength in their resilience, foster a nurturing environment for themselves and those they care for, and navigate the complexities of Alzheimer's with grace and compassion.

Honoring Memories

Creating meaningful rituals or tributes to celebrate and honor the life of the loved one can be a powerful aspect of coping with grief. This might involve ceremonies that reflect the individual's preferences and legacy, storytelling among family and friends to share and preserve memories, or creating a memorial tribute that captures their essence. These acts of remembrance serve as a testament to the love and bond shared, helping to keep the individual's spirit alive in the hearts of those who grieve.

Coping with grief and loss is an individualized and ongoing process, with no right or wrong way to navigate its complexities. It's essential for caregivers and loved ones to allow themselves the space and grace to mourn in their own time and manner, recognizing that grief can ebb and flow over time. By approaching this journey with patience, compassion, and self-kindness, individuals can find a path through grief that honors their loved one's memory and allows for healing and peace.

In providing end-of-life care for someone with Alzheimer's disease, the intertwining of compassion, empathy, and respect for the individual's dignity and wishes forms the foundation of genuinely supportive and meaningful care. Understanding the nuanced aspects of palliative and hospice care, managing symptoms with attentiveness and care, and navigating the emotional landscape of grief and loss are all integral to this profound caregiving journey.

Making End-of-Life Decisions

Making end-of-life decisions for individuals with Alzheimer's disease is a profound responsibility that involves deep reflection on the individual's wishes, values, and preferences for quality of life. These decisions are crucial to ensuring that care aligns with what the individual would have wanted, honoring their autonomy and dignity at a time when they may no longer be able to express their wishes directly.

Ethical Considerations

Ethical considerations are at the heart of making end-of-life decisions for individuals with Alzheimer's disease. They embody the moral complexities that caregivers and healthcare providers navigate in this delicate stage of care. The principles of beneficence, autonomy, and non-maleficence provide a framework for ethical decision-making, yet applying these principles in the context of advanced Alzheimer's involves nuanced judgment and deep compassion.

Assessing the individual's decision-making capacity becomes a cornerstone of ethical care. This involves carefully evaluating the person's ability to understand the implications of medical treatments and end-of-life care options. As cognitive impairment deepens, individuals may struggle to communicate their wishes. In such circumstances, advance directives become an invaluable guide, expressing the individual's preferences before their capacity is diminished. When advance directives are unavailable or specific situations are not addressed within them, the appointment of a healthcare proxy becomes essential. This designated individual, chosen for their understanding of the patient's values and wishes, assumes the responsibility of decision-making, striving to reflect what the individual would have chosen if they were able.

Considering the individual's quality of life is another critical ethical aspect. This includes a thoughtful evaluation of how various medical interventions align with the person's values, goals, and preferences for their remaining life. Decisions about life-sustaining treatments and palliative care options are made to maximize comfort, preserve dignity, and respect the individual's wishes to the fullest extent possible. It involves a delicate balance between extending life and enhancing the quality of the life that remains, often requiring difficult conversations about the benefits and burdens of continued medical intervention.

Respecting cultural and spiritual beliefs is integral to providing care that honors the whole person. Individuals may have deeply held beliefs that influence their preferences for end-of-life care, including decisions about specific treatments, rituals, and practices to be observed as they approach life's end. Understanding and integrating these beliefs into the care plan ensures that end-of-life care is medically appropriate and spiritually and culturally congruent with the individual's identity.

Facilitating shared decision-making involves creating a collaborative environment where family members, caregivers, and healthcare providers come together to discuss and decide on the best course of 0action. This process values open communication, ensuring all parties know the medical realities, potential outcomes, and ethical considerations. By building consensus, shared decision-making respects the autonomy of the individual with Alzheimer's while drawing on the collective wisdom and love of those who know them best.

In navigating the ethical complexities of end-of-life care for individuals with Alzheimer's disease, caregivers and healthcare providers are called to act with compassion, respect, and integrity. Balancing the principles of beneficence, autonomy, and non-maleficence requires a deep understanding of ethical frameworks and a heartfelt commitment to honoring the dignity and wishes of those facing the end of life. Through careful consideration of the individual's capacity, quality of life, cultural and spiritual beliefs, and the fostering of shared decision-making, ethical end-of-life care ensures that individuals are treated with the respect and love they deserve in their final days.

Communicating with Family Members

Effective communication within the family is a cornerstone of compassionate and respectful end-of-life decision-making for individuals with Alzheimer's disease. As caregivers navigate the complexities of care preferences, advance directives, and the myriad emotions accompanying these discussions, fostering an open, honest, and empathetic dialogue is essential. This approach ensures that the individual's wishes are honored and supports family unity and understanding during a profoundly challenging time.

Providing regular updates to family members is crucial in maintaining transparency about the individual's condition, treatment options, and any changes in their health status. These updates serve as a foundation for informed decision-making, ensuring that all family members are aware of the realities of the situation and can contribute to discussions from a place of understanding.

Encouraging open dialogue is equally important. Creating spaces where family members feel comfortable voicing their questions, concerns, and emotions fosters a sense of inclusion and respect. This open dialogue is essential for navigating the complexities of end-of-life care, where decisions often carry significant emotional weight and impact.

Respecting differing opinions among family members acknowledges the diversity of thought and feeling that characterizes human relationships. Recognizing that each family member may have their perspective on the best course of action underscores the importance of empathy and patience in these discussions. By valuing each voice, caregivers can facilitate a more harmonious decision-making process, even in disagreement.

Facilitating family meetings is a practical approach to ensuring all family members can be involved in decision-making. These in-person or virtual meetings provide a structured setting for discussing the individual's advance directives, treatment preferences, and any wishes they have expressed regarding end-of-life care. Family meetings offer a forum for collective reflection, discussion, and decision-making, reinforcing that end-of-life care is a shared journey.

Providing emotional support to family members is a compassionate acknowledgment of the emotional toll that making end-of-life decisions can take—recognizing and validating the grief, fear, and uncertainty that family members experience is essential to supportive caregiving. By offering reassurance, understanding, and empathy, caregivers can help family members navigate their emotional responses and foster a sense of collective resilience.

In conclusion, by prioritizing regular updates, encouraging open dialogue, respecting differing opinions, facilitating family meetings, and providing emotional support, caregivers can navigate the delicate process of making end-of-life decisions for individuals with Alzheimer's disease with dignity and respect. This comprehensive approach to communication helps ensure that decisions reflect the individual's wishes and values while also caring for the family's emotional well-being.

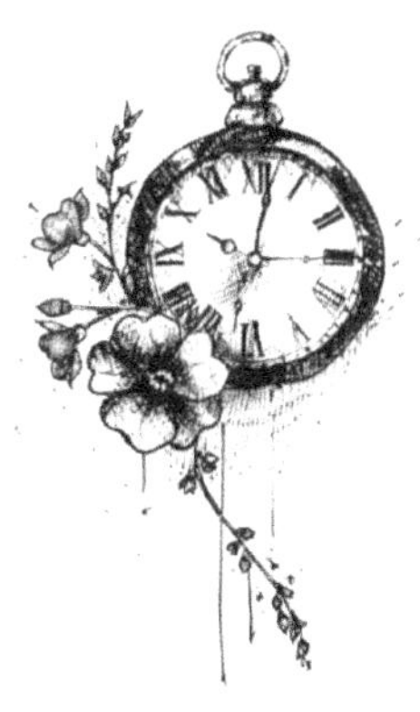

Conclusion

In the journey through this book, we have traversed the multifaceted landscape of Alzheimer's disease and the caregiving experience. From the initial diagnosis to the management of symptoms and through the legal and financial planning required to navigate this path, the book has aimed to equip readers with the knowledge and tools to provide compassionate care. Moreover, the emphasis on self-care for caregivers underscores the critical need for those providing support to attend to their well-being. The exploration of end-of-life care and decision-making has highlighted the importance of dignity and respect in the final stages of life.

Alzheimer's disease, with its progressive cognitive decline, memory loss, and behavioral changes, presents unique challenges that require a comprehensive approach to care. The management of symptoms through both pharmacological and non-pharmacological interventions is crucial for maintaining the quality of life for individuals with Alzheimer's. Equally important is addressing the legal and financial aspects of caregiving, ensuring that the needs and rights of both the caregiver and the person with Alzheimer's are protected and respected.

The role of self-care for caregivers cannot be overstated. In the demanding role of caregiving, caregivers need to prioritize their health and well-being, seeking support and utilizing respite care services to prevent burnout. Accessing resources, such as support groups and educational programs, provides caregivers with a support network and information critical to successfully navigating the caregiving journey.

Providing compassionate end-of-life care involves a deep understanding of the individual's preferences and values, ensuring that their final days are marked by dignity and comfort. This requires effective communication with family members and healthcare providers and a thoughtful consideration of ethical principles when making advance directives.

At the heart of caring for someone with Alzheimer's disease is the cultivation of compassion and empathy. Recognizing the inherent dignity and personhood of individuals with Alzheimer's is fundamental to providing care that honors their wishes and values. Caregivers are called to approach their role with understanding, patience, and respect, fostering a nurturing environment that supports the individual through the disease's challenges.

As we conclude this book, we recognize caregivers' profound journey, marked by challenges and moments of profound connection and understanding. For those seeking further information and support, a wealth of resources is available, from national organizations dedicated to Alzheimer's care to local support groups and online forums. These resources offer caregivers guidance, support, and community at every stage of their journey.

In navigating the complexities of Alzheimer's disease and caregiving, let us remember the power of compassion, empathy, and respect in transforming the caregiving experience. By embracing these values, caregivers can provide care that addresses the practical aspects of the disease and honors the deep human connection between caregiver and individual, making the journey a shared one filled with moments of love, understanding, and dignity.

As we reach the final chapter of my father's journey with Alzheimer's, it is with a heart whole of mixed emotions—grief for the loss that is to come, gratitude for the moments we shared, and a profound respect for the strength and dignity he maintained throughout his battle with this relentless disease. This chapter is not just a recounting of his last days but a tribute to the entirety of his life, the lessons he imparted, and the indelible mark he left on those who knew and loved him.

In the twilight of his journey, my father's world became smaller, the boundaries of his existence drawn ever tighter by the confines of Alzheimer's. Yet, within that space were moments of clarity and recognition, fleeting gifts that reminded us of the person he once was—a man of humor, intelligence, and profound kindness. Even in the silence, even as his memories faded, his essence, the core of who he was, remained a beacon for us to connect with.

Our conversations, once filled with stories of the past and plans for the future, became more straightforward. A squeeze of the hand, a smile, or a shared glance conveyed love and understanding that words could no longer express. We learned to communicate in the language of the heart, one that transcends the limitations of the mind.

We surrounded him with love in his final days, ensuring he was not alone. The room where he rested was filled with the sounds of his favorite music, photographs of cherished memories, and the presence of family and friends who came to say their goodbyes. It was a testament to the life he had lived and the impact he had on those around him.

I was with him at the end, holding his hand as he took his last breath. It was a peaceful passing, a gentle release from his struggles. At that moment, I felt an overwhelming sense of gratitude for our time together, the lessons he taught me, and his strength in facing Alzheimer's with grace and courage.

The final chapter of my father's life is not defined by the disease that took him from us but by the love, joy, and resilience he demonstrated throughout his life. It is a chapter of celebration, a reflection on the beauty of a life well-lived and the legacy of kindness, strength, and love he leaves behind. His journey with Alzheimer's taught us the true meaning of compassion, empathy, and the unbreakable bonds of family. It reminded us to cherish every moment, find joy in simple pleasures, and approach each day with love and gratitude.

As we close this chapter, we do so with hearts heavy with loss but also filled with love and memories that will endure. My father's journey has ended, but his spirit, lessons, and love live on in us. In remembering him, we honor his life, celebrate his legacy, and carry forward the light he brought into our lives.

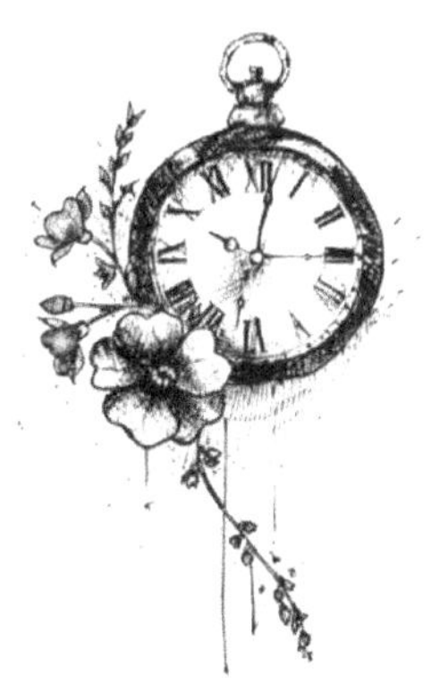

Resources

For readers who want to learn more about Alzheimer's disease and caregiving, the following resources may be helpful:

- Alzheimer's Association (https://www.alz.org/): This leading nonprofit organization is dedicated to Alzheimer's care, support, and research. It offers information, resources, and support services for individuals with Alzheimer's and their caregivers.
- Alzheimer's Society (https://www.alzheimers.org.uk/): A UK-based charity providing information, support, and resources for people living with dementia and their caregivers, including advice on diagnosis, treatment, and caregiving.
- National Institute on Aging – Alzheimer's and related Dementias Education and Referral Center (https://www.nia.nih.gov/health/alzheimers): A comprehensive resource from the National Institute on Aging offering information, research updates, and caregiving tips for Alzheimer's disease and related dementias.
- Caregiver Action Network (https://caregiveraction.org/): A nonprofit organization offering support, education, and resources for family caregivers, including tips, guides, and online communities for caregivers of individuals with Alzheimer's.

These resources provide valuable information, support, and guidance for individuals affected by Alzheimer's disease and their caregivers, empowering them to navigate the challenges of caregiving with knowledge, compassion, and resilience.

References

1. Alzheimer's Association - https://www.alz.org/

2. National Institute on Aging - https://www.nia.nih.gov/alzheimers

3. Mayo Clinic - https://www.mayoclinic.org/diseases-conditions/alzheimers-disease/symptoms-causes/syc-20350447

4. Alzheimer's Society - https://www.alzheimers.org.uk/

5. Alzheimer's Foundation of America - https://alzfdn.org/

6. WebMD - https://www.webmd.com/alzheimers/default.htm

7. Healthline - https://www.healthline.com/health/alzheimers-disease

8. Alzheimer's Research UK - https://www.alzheimersresearchuk.org/

9. Alzheimer's Disease Education and Referral Center - https://www.nia.nih.gov/health/alzheimers-disease-fact-sheet

10. Dementia Care Central - https://www.dementiacarecentral.com/

11. Alzheimer's Reading Room - https://alzheimersreadingroom.wordpress.com/

12. Caregiver Action Network - https://caregiveraction.org/

13. Alzheimer's Foundation of America - https://www.alzfdn.org/

14. Alzheimer's Research and Prevention Foundation - https://alzheimersprevention.org/

15. Family Caregiver Alliance - https://www.caregiver.org/

16. American Psychological Association - https://www.apa.org/topics/alzheimers

17. Johns Hopkins Medicine - https://www.hopkinsmedicine.org/health/conditions-and-diseases/alzheimers-disease

18. Alzheimer's & Dementia Weekly - https://www.alzheimersweekly.com/

Alzheimer's & Care Givers | Talking Therapy. https://www.talkingtherapyhondon.com/about-1-1/alzhiemers-care-givers

These references cover many reputable sources, including organizations, medical institutions, and support networks that provide valuable information and resources for understanding Alzheimer's disease, its stages, and caring for loved ones.